Speed Up & Sit Still

Martin Whitely, MLA, is married with two teenage sons. Before entering the Western Australian State Parliament in 2001 he worked as an accountant, university lecturer and high school teacher. He first became concerned about the use of ADHD medication by children in the 1990s, when he was alarmed at the number of medicated boys in his class. His advocacy is motivated solely by his experience as a teacher, parent and politician, and he has no commercial interests in ADHD treatments or products.

Martin Whitely

Speed Up & Sit Still

The Controversies of ADHD Diagnosis and Treatment

UWA PUBLISHING

First published in 2010 by
UWA Publishing
Crawley, Western Australia 6009
www.uwap.uwa.edu.au

UWAP is an imprint of UWA Publishing,
a division of The University of Western Australia

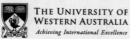

THE UNIVERSITY OF
WESTERN AUSTRALIA
Achieving International Excellence

Typeset in Bembo by J&M Typesetting
Printed by Griffin Press

National Library of Australia
Cataloguing-in-Publication entry:

Whitely, Martin.

Speed up and sit still : the controversies of ADHD diagnosis and treatment / Martin Whitely.

9781742582498 (pbk.)

Includes bibliographical references and index.

Attention-deficit hyperactivity disorder.
Attention-deficit hyperactivity disorder—Treatment.
Attention-deficit hyperactivity disorder—Diagnosis.

618.928589

Author royalties from this book will be donated by Martin Whitely to Drug Free Attention Difficulties Support Inc. (DFADS, www.dfads.org.) DFADS is a not-for-profit support group run by volunteers dedicated to helping parents with children experiencing atttentional difficulties.

Medical research has made such enormous advances that there are hardly any healthy people left.
ALDOUS HUXLEY

Introduction

Martin's ADHD Journey

I have always been competitive and, like most boys, prone to exaggerate my achievements. It is a fair boast, however, that from kindergarten until at least age fifteen I was the least organised, most distracted and least attentive boy in my year at school. I wasn't disobedient or exceptionally disruptive but I was an under-achieving daydreamer. My school reports always contained comments like 'Martin is totally disorganised and lacks concentration. With greater effort he could achieve much better results.' It wasn't because I had no interest in things academic. For a sporty kid I had a nerdish preoccupation with politics, current affairs and chess. Things that interested me demanded my attention; things that did not, did not.

For a few brief years as a senior at high school, I became more focused and achieved good academic results, way above anything I had previously managed. But then my early years at university were a disaster. Until I found the right formula for me of working full time with a heavy part-time study load, I lacked the motivation, pressure and focus to succeed. In truth it was only when I felt others expected me to fail that I was motivated to prove them wrong.

Eventually I graduated with a degree in accounting and after a few false starts in my mid-twenties I worked as an accountant. Although I had no difficulty understanding the theoretical foundations, I was a hopeless accountant because of my complete lack of interest in detail. I made the transition to teaching just before I turned thirty and found the challenge of educating, motivating and entertaining students exciting. Similarly, when I moved into politics in my early forties I found the diversity and constant pressure exhilarating.

As an accountant I was a square peg in a round hole. The constant movement and colour of teaching and politics are far better suited to my personality. I still lose things, am forgetful and distracted, have difficulty waiting my turn, occasionally fidget and sometimes 'self-medicate' with an excess of alcohol. However, at age fifty I have wonderfully happy work and home lives, structured in ways that cope with my weaknesses and build on my strengths.

I have no doubt that if I was born in 1999 and not 1959, I would be a candidate for a diagnosis of attention deficit hyperactivity disorder (ADHD). I have never considered myself diseased or disordered but I have completed internet-based self-assessment tests and been classed in the extreme ADHD range. The fact that children who behave like I once did are being classified as 'disordered' is why the focus of my political work has been advocating for distracted, impulsive, inattentive children.

I first heard of ADHD in 1995 when I began teaching at a wealthy independent boys grammar school and was struck by the number of 'medicated' students who seemed disengaged from their peers and unnaturally quiet and compliant. I had always considered that hyperactivity, impulsivity and disorganisation were part of what made boys boys. One student in particular alarmed me. Although Ted didn't appear to be a victim of bullying, he seemed to be almost completely isolated from his peers.[1] He was quiet and compliant, but seemed somehow 'absent'.

When set a forty-minute in-class essay Ted completed one sentence. I knew Ted had been diagnosed and medicated for ADHD and expected that, had the medication been working, he would have been able to produce more work. When I graded Ted's paper 'unsatisfactory' his parents arranged a meeting to 'educate' me about his condition. I sat quietly as Ted's father told me about Ted's biochemical brain imbalance and advised me to adjust my expectations of what Ted could achieve.

The next year as a fifteen-year-old, Ted went on a compulsory eleven-day hike with thirteen schoolmates and two female teachers. After the hike the teachers informed me that after a couple of days Ted's personality had transformed completely. He became a typically active, engaged and humorous teenage boy. These two strong-willed teachers' report on Ted's behaviour during the hike began: 'When Ted emerged from his drug-induced haze we saw a vibrant, interested, and interesting young man...' Of course the report was never sent to his parents, although they did request a meeting with the two teachers where they asked a number of questions: 'What happened on the hike? Ted can't stop talking about how wonderful it was. Were you aware that Ted forgot to take his ADHD medication that we had packed for him?' When the teachers suggested that the life-changing experience that Ted had on the hike may have been *because* he was medication-free, his parents disagreed, stating that Ted may have been able to function in a low-stress environment like hiking, but he could not possibly cope without medication at school.

I taught a number of other boys either on ADHD medication or for whom the pathway towards medication had been suggested. Often at the beginning of Year 11, where the academic rigour of subjects starts to see some students fall behind their peers, a checklist of ADHD behaviours would appear on my desk as part of the assessment process for a struggling student. For others, it was their cheeky demeanour and disinterest in an academic pathway that appeared to be the catalyst for an ADHD assessment. One boy diagnosed with, and medicated for, ADHD also had tics and Tourette syndrome, and frequently made involuntary and usually incomprehensible noises. At the time I thought the tics and Tourette syndrome were separate afflictions – years later I learned they were likely to have been side effects of his medication.

I was very uncomfortable with what I saw happening to these boys and frustrated at my inability to do anything about it. I remember attending a teachers professional development session at which a clinical psychologist informed us that the 5 per cent of the population who were the least attentive and most hyperactive had attention deficit hyperactivity disorder. The forty-minute presentation left me with an uneasy feeling that the science behind ADHD may not have been nearly as thorough as was made out. I thought the symptoms the psychologist identified – being disorganised, losing things and fidgeting – were pretty normal childhood behaviours and was uncomfortable with the idea of using drugs to control them.

From that point on I read widely on the issue. When I was a candidate for an unwinnable seat in the 1998 federal election, I decided to speak publicly, about my concerns about possible misdiagnosis and over-prescription of ADHD medications in an opinion piece in a local paper.

My activism on ADHD really kicked into gear when I was elected to the Western Australian Parliament in 2001. In my inaugural speech I spoke at length about the issue, confusing dexamphetamine and Ritalin, but nonetheless identifying 'my grave concerns that ADHD misdiagnosis and the resultant over-prescription of amphetamines' is 'a threat to the health and happiness of many West Australian children'.

For several years I was tentative with the language I used, believing that the medical profession must have had a solid scientific basis for its diagnosis of ADHD for at least some children. The more stories I heard and the more I researched the topic, however, the more suspicious I became – initially about the validity of the diagnosis, and then about the safety and efficacy of the drugs prescribed. The more evidence I was exposed to, the more suspicious I became about the motivation of those driving the widespread prescription of ADHD drugs. It's plain that the long-term use of amphetamines is bad for children, and the most puzzling part of the whole ADHD debate is how holding this position can be characterised as radical.

My decade-and-a-half-long journey through the ADHD debate has included many surprising twists and turns. The ADHD debate is like an onion: the more layers you peel away, the more you are inclined to cry.

1

Diagnosis: Disease, Disorder or Difference?

In 1987 a subcommittee of the American Psychiatric Association (APA), the majority of whose members had ties to the pharmaceutical industry, voted to include attention deficit hyperactivity disorder (ADHD) in the fourth edition of the *Diagnostic and Statistical Manual of Mental Disorders* (DSM-IV) the APA's catalogue of mental illness.[1] Similar processes had seen ADHD's predecessors attention deficit disorder (1980) and hyperactive disorder of children (1968) included in earlier editions of the DSM.

Every claim about ADHD should be viewed in the light of the diagnostic criteria defined in DSM-IV. In layman's terms, the diagnostic criteria for ADHD in all its forms results in the labelling of children who are too active (hyperactivity), not active enough (hypoactivity) and inattentive, as ADHD. The diagnosis of ADHD is entirely based on observations of a child's behaviour, as 'there are no laboratory tests, neurobiological assessments, or attentional assessments that have been established as diagnostic in the clinical assessment of Attention Deficit/ Hyperactivity Disorder'.[2]

Extract from DSM-IV: ADHD Diagnostic Criteria

Either (1) or (2):

1. six (or more) of the following symptoms of inattention have persisted for at least 6 months to a degree that is maladaptive and inconsistent with developmental level:

Inattention

   a. often fails to give close attention to details or makes careless mistakes in schoolwork, work, or other activities

   b. often has difficulty sustaining attention in tasks or play activities

   c. often does not seem to listen when spoken to directly

   d. often does not follow through on instructions and fails to finish schoolwork, chores, or duties in the workplace (not due to oppositional behavior or failure to understand instructions)

   e. often has difficulty organizing tasks and activities

   f. often avoids, dislikes, or is reluctant to engage in tasks that require sustained mental effort (such as schoolwork or homework)

   g. often loses things necessary for tasks or activities (e.g., toys, school assignments, pencils, books, or tools)

   h. is often easily distracted by extraneous stimuli

   i. is often forgetful in daily activities

2. six (or more) of the following symptoms of hyperactivity-impulsivity have persisted for at least 6 months to a degree

that is maladaptive and inconsistent with developmental level:

Hyperactivity
a. often fidgets with hands or feet or squirms in seat
b. often leaves seat in classroom or in other situations in which remaining seated is expected
c. often runs about or climbs excessively in situations in which it is inappropriate (in adolescents or adults, may be limited to subjective feelings of restlessness)
d. often has difficulty playing or engaging in leisure activities quietly
e. is often "on the go" or often acts as if "driven by a motor"
f. often talks excessively

Impulsivity
g. often blurts out answers before questions have been completed
h. often has difficulty awaiting turn
i. often interrupts or intrudes on others (e.g., butts into conversations or games)[3]

The eighteen behaviours are, according to ADHD proponents, evidence of a neurobiological disorder, that is, a 'biochemical brain imbalance', though most children, and many adults, display them to varying degrees in homes, schools and workplaces every day. Consider, too, that children are naturally impulsive, inquisitive, active, playful and often inattentive. The diagnostic criteria reflect very narrow expectations of what constitutes normality in young children. Television current affairs programs often portray ADHD children as violent, bad-tempered, uncontrollable brats, but the diagnostic criteria make no reference to violent or other extreme behaviours. Interrupting, talking excessively, being forgetful or not playing quietly are not extreme behaviours. They form a part of normal childhood behaviours and are not specific to ADHD. They also require that 'some hyperactive-impulsive or inattentive symptoms that cause impairment must have been present before age 7 years'.[4] Yet how many six-year-olds play quietly and await their turn patiently? Was childhood meant to be constrained, controlled, predictable and boring?

What is supposed to distinguish ADHD sufferers from the rest of the population is their level of behavioural impairment or dysfunction. Specifically, 'There must be clear evidence of clinically significant impairment in social, academic or occupational functioning' and 'Some impairment from the symptoms… present in two or more settings (e.g. at school or work and at home)'.[5] How 'often' a child 'fidgets or squirms in their seat', or 'interrupts' or 'avoids homework' or 'fails to remain seated when remaining seated is expected' or 'is distracted by external stimuli' so that they exhibit 'some impairment' is not defined in DSM–IV. Like beauty, 'impairment' is in the eye of the beholder. DSM–IV says:

> Signs of the disorder may be minimal or absent when the person is receiving frequent rewards for appropriate behaviour, is under close supervision, is in a novel setting, is engaged in especially interesting activities, or is in a one-to-one situation (e.g., the clinician's office.)[6]

In other words, ADHD children will behave appropriately and not display ADHD symptoms when they are rewarded, when people pay attention to them (close supervision) and when they are having new experiences. Conversely, ADHD children will be inattentive, easily distracted and display ADHD symptoms when their good behaviour goes unrewarded, no one pays any attention to them, or they are bored.

The diagnosing clinician doesn't have to observe any of the symptoms, let alone any impairment. He or she may simply base their diagnosis on third-party accounts of a child's behaviour. The child's parents and teachers usually provide these and are typically asked to fill in a questionnaire detailing if their child always, often, sometimes or never displays behaviour like avoiding homework and chores, losing toys, not listening, fidgeting, butting in, talking excessively or being easily distracted or forgetful.

Disturbingly, parents and teachers are rarely given guidance as to the crucial difference between sometimes and often. Even devoted parents, particularly first-time parents, can have unrealistic expectations of normal childhood behaviour. Nor is any guidance given to age-appropriate levels of attention or impulsivity control. The same imprecise, subjective diagnostic criteria are applied whether their child is two or seventeen.

What's of particular concern here is that parents and teachers are not routinely informed of the central role that their evidence plays in their child's diagnosis.

Many are simply fed the line that their child has a 'biochemical brain imbalance' – without any supporting evidence other than the observed behaviour of their child – and that this 'imbalance' is best treated with medication.

One counter argument to this is that all psychiatric disorders, many of which are also treated with medication, are diagnosed using similar behavioural criteria. Pointing out inadequacies in the diagnosis of other psychiatric conditions is a poor defence for the inadequacies of the ADHD diagnostic criteria. However, at least conditions like schizophrenia involve extreme behaviours such as delusions or catatonia.

Co-morbidity

DSM-IV makes no reference to a biochemical imbalance being the cause of ADHD, although it is treated as if it does have a single biochemical cause by the claim that, in the majority of cases, it is co-morbid — meaning that it co-exists with a range of other diseases and disorders.[7] Typically it's argued that the co-morbid conditions require separate but complementary treatments; in practice this means ADHD-specific drugs for ADHD and other drugs for co-morbid conditions. It is common for children to be on a range of drugs for bipolar disorder, depression, anxiety and ADHD simultaneously. South Australian psychiatrist Jon Jureidini rejects the concept of multiple co-morbid disorders: 'When you have got a kid with ADHD and oppositional defiance disorder and depression and anxiety disorder...what this says is not that he has got four disorders, but that there is something wrong with the kid and people haven't properly understood what it is yet.'[8]

Poor diet, sight, hearing, parenting, teaching, physical, sexual or psychological abuse or trauma, sedentary lifestyle, neurotoxin exposure, underlying medical conditions and even boredom can lead to a child failing to pay attention and/or acting in an impulsive or hyperactive manner. Most of these causes have little to do with 'brain chemistry'. Occasionally, however, neurotoxins may cause a biochemical imbalance in the brain and, if so, the source of the neurotoxins should be identified and removed. The use of drugs to address a biochemical brain imbalance caused by toxins simply introduces yet another toxin.

Jon Jureidini believes the rise in ADHD prescribing is caused in part by doctors who jump too quickly to unwarranted conclusions, stating: 'If you are going to be a good psychiatrist or a good mental [health] professional you have to be able to tolerate that [vast] level of uncertainty and not go grasping for the prescription pad or the MRI scan or whatever the latest fad is to deal with that complicated issue.'[9]

Jureidini also believes that in some cases abuse or neglect may be 100 per cent responsible for children's errant behaviour while with other cases parenting has very little to do with it. The diagnosis of ADHD and subsequent medicating of children can hide serious child abuse. It's obvious, for example, that children who have been sexually or physically abused are highly likely to be inattentive and behave inappropriately. I recall a phone call from a woman whose nine-year-old grand-daughter had been a victim of sustained sexual abuse by a family member. She was distraught that her daughter had allowed the young girl to be medicated for ADHD. On dexamphetamine (a psychostimulant) her grand-daughter had become quiet and withdrawn, which apparently pleased her mother, but exasperated the grandmother who believed her real issues were being masked by medication. Severely traumatised children are likely to avoid homework, be easily distracted, lose things, fidget and squirm. Victorian child psychiatrist Dr George Halasz believes medicating an abused child further damages that child's self-esteem: 'If a child victim of abuse is diagnosed with ADHD and medicated, it will break all their trust in relationships. They perceive themselves as damaged goods.'[10]

The History of ADHD

In 1902 Dr Fredric Still documented cases involving impulsiveness, labelling it a 'defect of moral control'. It was later renamed 'minimal brain damage'. In 1922 the symptoms were further defined and given the name 'post encephalitic behaviour disorder'.

The use of stimulants to modify behaviour did not begin until 1937 when American doctor Charles Bradley was the first to recommend stimulants to treat hyperactive children. Dr Bradley

> observed the 'calming' effect of stimulants on children when he gave Benzedrine (trademark for amphetamine) to a group of 30 children in order to treat headaches that resulted from spinal taps they were given. The Benzedrine did not do anything for the headaches, but it did make the children less active and more compliant, in a fashion he called 'spectacular'.[11]

Bradley had identified the effects of amphetamines on 'normal' children but proposed amphetamines as a treatment for hyperactive children. In 1950 Dr Bradley undertook a study of 275 hyperactive children given amphetamines. He reported 'between 60 per cent and 70 per cent to be much improved while on the drugs'.[12]

And in 1956 the stimulant Ritalin made its first appearance in the treatment of these hyperactive children. Despite these early origins it was not until well into the 1960s that the use of stimulant medication to treat hyperactive children became common, and not until the 1990s that, facilitated by the loosening of the DSM-IV diagnostic criteria, prescribing rates exploded in North America and Australia.[13]

Except for Still's 'defects of moral control', early emphasis was on aetiology-based (cause) descriptions of the disorder. This is despite the fact that the cause or causes had never been established. The term 'minimal brain dysfunction' used in the early 1960s was altered in the late 1970s to 'hyperactive disorder of childhood'. This name change drastically altered public perception of the disorder. No one wanted to have a brain-damaged child – having a hyperactive child was far more acceptable.

During the 1970s, further symptoms such as a lack of focus and daydreaming were added to the diagnostic list. Impulsiveness was also expanded at this time to include verbal, cognitive and motor impulsiveness. In 1980 the APA voted to change the name of the disorder to 'attention deficit disorder' (ADD) and its definition was again expanded. The new definition was based on the assumption that attention difficulties are sometimes independent of impulse problems and hyperactivity – the disorder was redefined as primarily a problem of inattention, rather than of hyperactivity. In keeping with this approach, two subtypes of ADD were presented in DSM-III: ADD/H, with hyperactivity, and ADD/WO, without hyperactivity or passive ADD. The recognition of passive ADD has been the subject of debate ever since.

Passive ADHD

When the third edition of the *Diagnostic and Statistical Manual of Mental Disorders* (DSM-IIIR) was revised in 1987, the name of the condition was changed to the one we use today, attention deficit hyperactivity disorder (ADHD), and the symptoms were again merged into a single disorder without any subtypes. Specifically, DSM-IIIR required a child to display six of nine inattentive behaviours *and* six of nine impulsive/hyperactive behaviours. This diagnostic requirement did away with the possibility that an individual could have the disorder without being hyperactive. A child had to display both inattentive and hyperactive/impulsive behaviours.

Subsequent to the release of DSM-IIIR a number of studies were published justifying the existence of passive or inattentive ADD without the hyperactivity element. In response to this backlash, the definition was changed yet again in the fourth edition of the manual published in 1994 (DSM-IV). The criteria was broadened so that a child needed to display six of nine inattentive *or* six of nine hyperactive/impulsive behaviours. The APA did not change the name ADHD, but the symptoms were divided into two categories: inattentive and hyperactive/impulsive. Three subtypes of the disorder were also defined: 'ADHD – Primarily Inattentive', 'ADHD – Primarily Hyperactive/Impulsive', and 'ADHD – Combined Type (both inattentive and impulsive)'. Not surprisingly, this created some confusion. (Sometimes when the term ADD is used today it is used in its original generic sense – interchangeably with ADHD. On other occasions it is a specific descriptor of passive ADHD.)

ADHD now applies to a whole spectrum of child behaviour. Both children who are too active and children who are too inactive are included. In addition to the ADHD hyperactive and inattentive subtypes, DSM-IVTR, the updated version of DSM-IV contains yet another category, 'Attention Deficit/ Hyperactivity Disorder – Not otherwise specified', which further broadens the criteria to include 'individuals whose symptom pattern does not meet the full criteria for the disorder'.

Fred Baughman, American neurologist and author of *The ADHD Fraud*, believes this broadening of diagnostic criteria is contrary to the process of defining legitimate diseases. In 2006 Baughman wrote:

> Normally, as a condition is studied and more is learned about it, the diagnostic signs (signs=objective abnormalities) are narrowed down to a specific set of objective criteria that can be reliably applied. With ADHD the opposite happened…[14]

With the benefit of hindsight, Dr Allen Frances, who was the chief of psychiatry at the Duke University Medical Center and led the effort to update DSM-IV in 1994, regretted broadening the diagnostic criteria and warned of problems with the drafting of the next edition, DSM-V, due for final release in 2012. Frances believes:

We learned some very, very, painful lessons in doing DSM IV...we thought we were being really careful about everything we did and we wanted to discourage changes. But inadvertently, I think we helped to trigger three false epidemics. One for Autistic Disorder... another for the childhood diagnosis of Bi-Polar Disorder and the third for the wild over-diagnosis of Attention Deficit Disorder.[15]

Significant effort has been put into promoting and normalising passive ADHD in the public realm, much of it centred on the argument that girls were being underdiagnosed as they were more likely to have passive ADHD than exhibit hyperactivity. Typical of this is the following extract published in the *West Australian*, 16 April 2003.

Quiet Children Slip ADHD Net

Children with attention deficit disorders who are not naughty and disruptive are falling through the medical net, resulting in learning difficulties and social problems, according to a WA expert. Curtin University psychology professor, David Hay, who specialises in attention deficit hyperactivity disorder, said children with a form of the disorder that makes them dreamy and inattentive were often not diagnosed until their teens if at all. Girls were most likely to slip through the net. The form of ADHD most widely known – when children are noisy and difficult – was more common in boys but both boys and girls were equally likely to have 'quiet' ADHD.

'ADHD is meant to be diagnosed by the age of seven but with a lot of girls, it only comes to the fore when they get to high school,' Professor Hay said. 'It becomes obvious in high school

> because they are no longer in just one class, they have to move classes all the time and be organised, so all the organisational problems with ADHD suddenly come to the fore. When we did surveys in schools, about 4 per cent to 5 per cent of kids have this inattentive type (of ADHD) but because they are quiet kids no one really picks it up...[16]

Adult ADHD

Many parents take the advice that ADHD is inheritable at face value and become suspicious that they may share the 'lifelong affliction' with their child. The subsequent diagnosis of adult ADHD is in their minds confirmed when they become temporarily more focused after taking medication. DSM-IV says: 'Some hyperactive-impulsive or inattentive symptoms that caused impairment were present before age 7 years.' Despite this and the fact that the diagnostic criteria are defined in terms most applicable to children in a classroom setting, in recent years considerable energy has been put into promoting 'Adult ADHD'.

The Western Australian ADHD support group, the Learning and Attentional Disorders Society (LADS) (see chapter 3), attributes a variety of adult problems from car crashes to divorce and even bad manners to undiagnosed Adult ADHD:

> The symptoms of ADHD can cause severe disruptions in the lives of adults: Concentration difficulties may result in people becoming procrastinators, and earning a reputation for laziness and a lack of motivation. They may be embarrassed in social situations as their

concentration drifts during conversations. They may have a tendency to interrupt others or to make tactless comments. Physically, they may engage in high-risk activities. People with ADHD receive more traffic infringements and licence suspensions, particularly for speeding. They are involved in more motor vehicle accidents. Intimate relationships may be more difficult to sustain, with higher rates of separation and divorce occurring in this group. Educational and professional under-achievement is common, and causes great frustration. Adults with ADHD often find it difficult to manage their ADHD children...Dexamphetamine and Methylphenidate improve symptoms in up to 78 per cent of adults with ADHD.[17]

Even criminality and drug abuse are attributed to undiagnosed, and therefore un-medicated, ADHD. An example is the following verbal evidence given on behalf of LADS to the 2004 Western Australian parliamentary inquiry into ADHD:

The research shows that people with ADHD are six times more likely to develop a substance abuse problem. However, if they are treated with stimulant medication, the risk is reduced to the same as someone without ADHD...Some excellent work has been done by Dr Tony Mastrioni on the New South Wales prison system. He estimates that 30 per cent of the prison population in NSW has ADHD, either diagnosed or undiagnosed.[18]

The effect of this association with extreme dysfunctional behaviour is to create a sense of crisis that extreme consequences will result from ADHD going untreated which really means un-medicated.

Criminal and drug-taking behaviour are in themselves dysfunctional and most often impulsive acts. How many drug addicts aren't forgetful, distracted or disorganised? It is self-evident that many criminals and drug addicts tend to demonstrate ADHD behaviours and certainly live dysfunctional lives, therefore qualifying for a diagnosis of adult ADHD. Yet to argue that ADHD, when left un-medicated, causes criminal behaviour or drug abuse is to confuse cause and effect. It involves identifying dysfunction in what is already identified as a dysfunctional population. This is the equivalent of being able to bet on a horse after the race has finished.

Consensus As a Substitute for Science

Consensus rather than science has driven the expansion of the definition of ADHD. In 2002, an 'independent consortium' of eighty-four 'leading scientists' signed the 'International Consensus Statement on ADHD'. The first signatory was the world's high profile ADHD advocate, American psychologist Dr Russell Barkley.

Extract from the 'International Consensus Statement on ADHD'

This is the first consensus statement issued by an independent consortium of leading scientists concerning the status of the disorder. Among scientists who have devoted years, if not entire careers, to the study of this disorder there is no controversy regarding its existence...We cannot over emphasize the point that, as a matter of science, the notion that ADHD does not exist is simply wrong...the occasional coverage of the disorder casts the story in the form of a sporting event with evenly matched competitors. The views of a handful of non-expert doctors that ADHD does not exist are contrasted against mainstream scientific views that it does, as if both views had equal merit. Such attempts at balance give the public the impression that there is substantial scientific disagreement over whether ADHD is a real medical condition. In fact, there is no such disagreement – at least no more so than there is over whether smoking causes cancer, for example, or whether a virus causes HIV/AIDS...To publish stories that ADHD is a fictitious disorder or merely a conflict between today's Huckleberry Finns and their caregivers is tantamount to declaring the earth flat, the laws of gravity debatable, and the periodic table in chemistry a fraud...All of the major medical associations and government health agencies recognize ADHD as a genuine disorder because the scientific evidence indicating it is so is overwhelming.[19]

The claim that the signatories were an 'independent consortium' is questionable on a number of levels. First, there is the obvious investment in validating the authenticity of a controversial disorder for those 'who have devoted years, if not entire careers' to its study. In addition, many of the self-appointed consortium of 'leading scientists' earn their incomes either through diagnosing and prescribing for ADHD or conducting drug-company funded research into the 'disorder'.

It is the widespread acceptance of ADHD by 'the major medical associations and government health agencies' that is the most alarming part of the whole debate. Here, hypothesis is stated as fact and, in the minds of many, ADHD is so big it *must* be real. Few people in the medical and political establishment are motivated enough to examine the quality of the research or brave enough to question the validity of the diagnosis.

British psychiatrist Sami Timimi believes the Consensus Statement was a response to the authors being 'shaken by criticism' of ADHD diagnosing and prescribing.[20] Timimi is highly critical of the Consensus Statement and sees it as an attempt to shut down debate:

> Not only is it completely counter to the spirit and practice of science to cease questioning the validity of ADHD as proposed by the consensus statement, there is an ethical and moral responsibility to do so. It is regrettable that they wish to close down debate prematurely and in a way not becoming of academics. The evidence shows that the debate is far from over.[21]

The authors of the Consensus Statement, according to Timimi, 'are well-known advocates of drug treatment for children with ADHD' who in the statement did 'not declare their financial interests and/or their links with pharmaceutical companies'.[22]

The International Consensus Statement is an attempt by its authors to present the legitimacy of ADHD as an indisputable truth. Documents such as this have the effect of dumbing down debate by substituting prejudice for science. Despite the fundamentalist fervour of the authors, the fact is that ADHD is no more than a very loosely defined set of symptoms for which self-appointed 'leading scientists' identify no cure.

The Question of Difference

Most of the research undertaken by proponents of ADHD, including the signatories of the International Consensus Statement, is designed to show that ADHD medication works or that children diagnosed with ADHD are different from other children. The many claims of new research purporting to prove this difference, however, have been shown to be false. Many of the studies that claim to show differences compared brains that had never been medicated to brains that had been exposed to psychostimulants. Psychostimulants 'routinely cause gross malfunctions in the brain of the child' and 'can cause shrinkage (atrophy) or other permanent physical abnormalities'.[23] Most of the supposed breakthroughs relate to brain-imaging using PET scanners or MRI technology. None of the claims, however, have been sustained and all mainstream medical authorities recognise that the technologies have no role in the diagnosis of ADHD. Even the more optimistic of assessments recognise brain-imaging technologies as having no diagnostic value, merely unfulfilled potential.[24] Neuro-imaging can do little more than assess the shape and size of the brain.[25] Queensland psychologist Bob

Jacobs believes:

> even if researchers found a consistent difference between children who act a certain way ('ADHD') and children who don't, and even if they could some-how prove that the difference caused the behaviours, there is no reason to believe there is any 'disorder'. There may be physiological differences between people who are right-handed and left-handed, or people who prefer the colour red over the colour blue. But it doesn't make either group 'sick'. We know that people have individual physical differences, but it is dangerous ground to say that those differences are a 'disorder', just because they are in the minority, or because the cause problems with fitting into society's rigid structures (like school).[26]

As Jacobs points out, the search for differences in ADHD brains, which has so far proven fruitless, is also futile. For even if the search was eventually successful, all it could demonstrate is difference, not disease.

Prevalence Rates

Prevalence rates are estimates of the percentage of a population with a disease or disorder. A prevalence rate is different from a diagnosis rate, which is the percentage of the population diagnosed with a condition. For diseases like asthma, haemophilia, or leukaemia – with science-based diagnoses, real and indisputable negative consequences, and medically valid treatments – parents, policymakers and clinicians need to be concerned if prevalence rates exceed diagnosis rates because it means that real disease is going undiagnosed and therefore untreated. For a subjective, ill-defined diagnosis like ADHD, estimates of prevalence rates are virtually meaningless. Even if levels of inattention, hyperactivity and impulsivity could be objectively measured so children could be reliably placed on a continuum of ADHD behaviours, that would not make it a legitimate disorder.

In spite of this inability to objectively measure an ultimately meaningless statistic, estimates of prevalence rates are frequently quoted. They are used to defend allegations that ADHD is over-diagnosed and over-medicated with the claim that prevalence rates exceed diagnosis and prescribing rates and that ADHD is in fact *under*-diagnosed and *under*-medicated. There have been numerous studies to determine prevalence rates for ADHD. Not surprisingly, estimates of ADHD prevalence vary widely. An American study conducted in 1998 found that prevalence estimates vary between 1.7 per cent and 16 per cent.[27] Estimates of prevalence rates also vary across cultures, presumably influenced by cultural norms with the highest reported (29 per cent) being in India.[28] The huge range is undoubtedly a consequence of relying on subjective and ill-defined diagnostic criteria.

11.2 per cent NHMRC Prevalence Estimate

The National Health and Medical Research Council (NHMRC) is an independent statutory agency funded by the Commonwealth government to develop recommendations for best health policy and practice. In 2000, research outsourced by the NHMRC estimated that 11.2 per cent of Australian children had ADHD.[29] The methodology used in the study was fundamentally flawed. It involved the parents of 2737 children completing a checklist on the behaviour of their child,[30] not an effort to ensure the children being tested met the full criteria for a diagnosis of ADHD. There was no measure for impairment or any attempt to establish that the child displayed the behaviours in at least two settings, nor were other explanations for the ADHD type behaviours explored.

As a result the 11.2 per cent estimate was a gross overestimate of the number of Australian children who would qualify for a thorough application of the DSM–IV criteria. A prevalence of 11.2 per cent equates to one in nine Australian children. It is widely accepted that ADHD is far more common in boys than in girls at a ratio of approximately three to one.[31] Given that ratio and assuming a prevalence rate of 11.2 per cent, one in six boys, and one in eighteen girls would have ADHD medication. A stunning and frightening prospect. Nonetheless, this study has been frequently used to support the argument that ADHD is under-diagnosed and under-medicated. One of many examples of this abuse of statistics was by former president of the Western Australian AMA Dr Bernard Pearn-Rowe, who in 2002 was quoted as saying, '[in Western Australia] local specialists were leading the way in diagnosing and treating the condition…a 1999 review by the National Health and Medical Research Council found 11 per cent of the population aged 4 to 17 years had ADHD, but that less than 2 per cent of cases were treated'.[32] The fact that a state leader of the AMA unquestioningly accepted this advice is evidence of a deficit of common sense at the highest levels of the Western Australian medical fraternity.

Of much greater concern is that in November 2009, nearly a decade after the flawed estimate was produced, federal health minister Nicola Roxon, the Royal Australasian College of Physicians and the NHMRC used the 11.2 per cent estimate, in a joint press release, to claim there were over 350,000 Australian children and adolescents with ADHD.[33] It is extremely worrying that old, specious, discredited research can be recycled by the highest levels of government and the medical profession.

2

Amphetamine Deficit Disorder

Applying the label 'ADHD' to a range of childhood behaviours implies it has a common cause. ADHD, really just a collection of loosely defined behavioural symptoms, is mistakenly regarded as the biological cause. Psychologist and Professor Emeritus at California State University, David Keirsey, criticises the circularity of the argument stating, 'It's preposterous to say that the symptoms of attention deficit cause the deficit of attention.'[1]

The obvious way to fix a biochemical problem is to use a biochemical solution – medication. There is no doubt that medication is the most immediate method of altering behaviour. There is also no doubt that extreme ADHD-type behaviours can be problematic; however, medication simply masks these symptoms and does nothing to address underlying causes.

In short-term research trials pharmacological interventions invariably appear more effective than non–drug treatments for two reasons. First, drugs alter behaviour much faster than non-drug treatments, and trials most often measure improvements by short-term symptom management (often for no longer than a few weeks). Second, while the behaviour-altering effects of stimulants are almost universal, other forms of treatment are not. Family counselling, for example, will be of little or no benefit if the underlying cause of behavioural problems is exposure to environmental toxins.

In many cases there is nothing to 'treat'. Many children are naturally inattentive, impulsive and hyperactive. In these cases normal childhood behaviour is pathologised and healthy children are 'medicated'. Perhaps subconsciously for many busy, stressed adults, being able to control their child's challenging behaviour is their main concern. If so, stimulant medication wins hands down.

The Effects of Amphetamines

The most commonly used drugs to treat ADHD are the amphetamine-based psychostimulants dexamphetamine (current brand names Adderall, Dexedrine, Dexostrat) and methylphenidate (Ritalin, Concerta, Attenta).[2] Their stimulant effects are very short, lasting a matter of hours with 'no evidence that the medications promote or cause psychological, social, or emotional growth' in the long term.[3] The temporary effects of medication create the illusion of a solution to challenging and inconvenient behaviours. It is as if the deficit of attention was caused by a deficit of amphetamines. With the drugs in their system ADHD children are regarded as 'balanced'; without them they are considered faulty.

The effects of medicinal amphetamines are virtually indistinguishable from illicit ones. In the US prescription speed, i.e. methamphetamine (brand name Desoxyn), is used as an ADHD treatment. Speed and cocaine when taken orally in low doses have similar temporary 'performance enhancing' effects to dexamphetamine and Ritalin. With a therapeutic dose of stimulants in their system most people become more compliant. This, in the minds of many parents, is evidence that their child's 'biochemical imbalance' has been balanced.

When the the drugs wear off, however, there are often 'bounce' or withdrawal effects that worsen ADHD-type behaviours. Indeed, 'rebound' or withdrawal effects can occur that are 'often worse than the child's original or "baseline" behaviour', even after a single dose.[4] In 1978 a placebo controlled, double-blind study found over 70 per cent of 'normal children' aged six to twelve, given one typical therapeutic dose of stimulants, exhibited 'a marked behavioural rebound…starting approximately 5 hours after medication had been given; this consisted of excitability, talkativeness, and, for three children, apparent euphoria.'[5] Although in this study the 'normal children' exhibited the 'overactivity' symptoms of ADHD, the rebound effect can vary markedly 'from excitement to exhaustion and hypersomnia (excessive sleeping)'.[6] Witnessing the rebound effect reinforces parents' and teachers' belief that the child is chemically imbalanced without the drug and that he or she needs to keep taking medication. The pharmaceutical companies benefit from the rebound effect their products have created, to their great profit. They now have a customer with an ongoing 'need' for their product.

The American Psychiatric Association has long understood

the indiscriminate effect of amphetamines. In 1996 Dr Debra Zarin, representing the APA and the American Academy of Child and Adolescent Psychiatry, testified to a US Congressional committee that:

> It is a commonly held misconception that if a stimulant calms a child, that he must have ADHD; if he didn't have the disorder, the thinking goes, the medication would not have any effect. That is not true. Stimulants increase attention span in normal children as well as those with ADHD.[7]

American paediatrician and academic Dr Lydia Furman agrees, expressing concern that the use of stimulants as a diagnostic trial has the capacity to be a self-fulfilling prophecy:

> The use of stimulant medications in children with symptoms of hyperactivity and inattention is promoted by some as a diagnostic trial. The working plan is that if the child looks, acts, or functions better on a stimulant medication, then he or she should be on the medication, and a diagnosis of ADHD has been confirmed. However, studies have shown that behavioural response to stimulants does not distinguish children with diagnosed ADHD from normal children; thus, a behavioural response does not constitute either a diagnosis or a treatment but rather an expected response to medication.[8]

Performance Enhancers or Creativity Crushers?

Many critics of ADHD medications acknowledge their performance-enhancing properties. In July 2004 child psychiatrist Dr George Halasz said, 'Amphetamines are a performance enhancer, that's why students take them to study and truck drivers take them for concentration.'[9] However, the world's most prominent ADHD critic, New York psychiatrist Dr Peter Breggin, considers this narrowing of a child's focus an adverse reaction. Breggin cites extreme cases of children displaying obsessive-compulsive behaviours such as playing the same game over and over again or exhausting themselves performing repetitive tasks like raking up leaves, and he describes one case where a boy waits under the tree for a leaf to fall.[10] He argues that increased obedience to routine instructions may temporarily benefit other students, teachers and even parents, but is not evidence of improved functionality of the child, particularly when it comes at the expense of creativity.

Perhaps the key distinction between ADHD sceptics and ADHD proponents is their tolerance of difference. High-profile signatory of the 'International Consensus Statement on ADHD', Dr Russell Barkley (see chapter 1), agrees that compliance is often achieved through the use of drugs.[11] The difference, however, is that Dr Barkley regards non-compliance as a problem and Dr Breggin does not: 'Although inattention, overactivity, and poor impulse control are the most common symptoms cited by others as primary in hyperactive children, my own work with these children suggests that non-compliance is also a primary problem.'[12] There is something distinctly Orwellian in regarding a lack of compliance as a problem that warrants medicating. It is as if defective products (children) need balancing to achieve minimum quality control standards.

As well as valuing compliance Dr Barkley appears unconcerned that psychostimulants reduce a child's interest in social interactions. In 1979 he authored a study confirming the effect, writing, 'it has been reported that stimulant drugs reduce the child's interest in social interactions. Several observations in this study would support this notion.'[13] I saw this effect among numerous medicated boys in my classroom and in contrast to Dr Barkley regard this lack of social interaction as unacceptable and dehumanising. Dr Breggin has described this lack of interest in peer interactions and unnatural compliance as the 'zombie effect'.[14]

Addiction and Abuse

The 'zombie effect' is fairly minor when compared to many of the other potentially life-threatening side effects of ADHD stimulants. In 1995 the US Drug Enforcement Agency (DEA) warned that Ritalin use 'may be a risk factor for substance abuse'.[15] Even the inventors of ADHD, the American Psychiatric Association recognise that amphetamines, methylphenidate and cocaine are 'neuro-pharmacologically alike'.[16] The fourth edition of the *Diagnostic and Statistical Manual of Mental Disorders* recognises the abuse and addiction of these drugs in a common class of 'Amphetamine or Amphetamine-Like – Related Disorders'. It states: 'Prescribed stimulants have sometimes been diverted into the illegal market...Most of the effects of amphetamines and amphetamine-like drugs are similar to those of cocaine.'[17] Furthermore, the diagnostic criteria for 'Amphetamine Intoxication' include 'recent use of amphetamine or a related substance (e.g. methylphenidate)' and many of their potential side effects such as 'impaired social or occupational functioning, tachycardia, elevated blood pressure, nausea or vomiting, weight loss dyskinesias and dystonia'.[18] All ADHD stimulants are addictive and carry similar warnings for abuse.[19]

Extract from Prescribing Information for Dexedrine (a brand of dexamphetamine)

AMPHETAMINES HAVE A HIGH POTENTIAL FOR ABUSE. ADMINISTRATION OF AMPHET-AMINES FOR PROLONGED PERIODS OF TIME MAY LEAD TO DRUG DEPENDENCE AND MUST BE AVOIDED. PARTICULAR ATTENTION SHOULD BE PAID TO THE POSSIBILITY OF SUBJECTS OBTAINING AMPHETAMINES FOR NON-THERAPEUTIC USE OR DISTRIBUTION TO OTHERS, AND THE DRUGS SHOULD BE PRESCRIBED OR DISPENSED SPARINGLY.

MISUSE OF AMPHETAMINES MAY CAUSE SUDDEN DEATH AND SERIOUS CARDIO-VASCULAR ADVERSE EVENTS.

Parents and patients rely on prescribing clinicians to heed such warnings, or, at the very least, pass them on and inform them of the risks.

In 1998 Perth parents Mick and Val Murray took their

twelve-year-old daughter Claire Murray to a paediatrician. She was diagnosed with ADHD and put on 40 milligrams of dexamphetamine a day. Tragically Claire went on to develop an addiction to amphetamines and then heroin, and caught hepatitis B through needle sharing. Her liver failed and she received a transplant in 2009. Within months of receiving the transplant Claire returned to abusing heroin and her donated liver failed. Mick and Val Murray attribute Claire's addiction to her introduction to dexamphetamine. They told me on three occasions they were never informed about the addictive nature of dexamphetamine.[20] In 2010 Claire's case became highly publicised when the Western Australian government provided a $250,000 interest-free loan to her family so that she could undergo a live liver transplant in Singapore. Claire's aunt Caroline courageously provided a partial liver donation and in March 2010 Claire and her aunt were operated on in Singapore. Sadly, Claire's second transplant failed due to complications, and she died aged twenty-five in Singapore on 1 April 2010, surrounded by Mick, Val and other family members, but away from her two young children.

Perth: A Case History of Amphetamine Abuse

Despite the clear warnings and the tragic reality of many teenagers such as Claire Murray, one of the most aggressively marketed claims about ADHD is that its 'under-recognition' is a cause of illicit drug abuse. It is argued that early identification of ADHD and subsequent medication prevents undiagnosed individuals using illicit drugs to self-medicate.[21] (See also chapter 1.)

In the 1990s and early 2000s Western Australia, particularly Perth, had Australia's highest ADHD amphetamine prescription rate. If the above claims about drug abuse were correct, it would be expected that corresponding rates of abuse be among the lowest in Australia. The evidence suggests the opposite. When WA had Australia's highest dexamphetamine prescription rate, it also had the highest amphetamine abuse rates and relatively high rates of abuse for other illicit drugs.[22]

In 1999 illicit amphetamine abuse rates among secondary school children were the highest in the nation, over double the national average. Abuse rates for cannabis, tranquillisers, steroids, cocaine, ecstasy, heroin and LSD/hallucinogenics were all above the national average.[23] When Perth's prescribing rates for children plummeted so did amphetamine abuse rates. Between 2002 and 2008 there was a 51 per cent reduction (for people aged twelve to seventeen years).[24] This massive decline occurred at the same time as a huge fall (60 to 70 per cent) in child prescribing rates. (See also chapter 6.) This evidence is unequivocal; it clearly supports the commonsense proposition that prescribing amphetamines facilitates their abuse.

Even though abuse rates began to drop by 2005, a survey of Western Australian secondary school students (the Australian School Students Alcohol and Drug Survey or ASSAD) found that 84 per cent of those who had abused amphetamines in the last year had abused prescription amphetamines.[25] The same survey found that 27 per cent of twelve- to seventeen-year-olds who had been prescribed stimulant medication either gave it away or sold it.[26] The survey also showed that 45 per cent of students who had ever taken dexamphetamine or methylphenidate were not prescribed the drugs by a doctor.[27] Unfortunately, similar statistics are not collected when the ASSAD survey is conducted in other states. Giving subsidised amphetamines to teenagers obviously carries a considerable risk that they will abuse, or provide or sell them to others. This risk is naturally increased for teenagers identified as exhibiting dysfunctional, impulsive behaviour.

The diversion of ADHD amphetamines has significant policy implications. The Commonwealth government spends tens of millions of dollars annually subsidising them through the Pharmaceutical Benefits Scheme. When they are diverted for illicit use, the Commonwealth government unwittingly becomes a major sponsor of amphetamine abuse. This connection, well understood by Perth teenagers of the 1990s, is completely overlooked by Commonwealth legislators and policy makers removed from the reality of prescription amphetamine diversion.

Coming Down
by Clare Trevelyan

The enormous supply of the ADHD medication dexamphetamine or dexies as we call them was [we thought] the best thing to ever happen to us at high school. I went to Hollywood Senior High School in Nedlands and graduated in 2000. Everyone knew what dexies were: some kids were prescribed, some bought them, some sold them, some took them recreationally and some took them to study. And all up the train lines, from Fremantle to Joondalup, kids had bottles of dexies rattling around in their backpacks. You'd be hard pressed to find a teenager who didn't know what they were and, from nerds to the junkies, from Presbyterian Ladies College to Balga Senior High, everyone took them.

From what I have seen, they are still very popular today. Why? First because the amphetamine keeps you up all night, and second because you can get it for a fraction of the price of speed, from a doctor. But mostly, because it simply makes you feel good.

For those of you who have never tried dexies, I will explain what it feels like. After about 30 minutes of taking two or three tablets, you begin to feel as though you could do almost anything. Your heart rate increases and you can work, talk or read for hours on end with no need for a break, all the while feeling great about whatever it is you are doing. You may scrape your lips with your teeth a little too often, talk rapidly, but other than that show no outward signs of being 'on drugs'.

The amount of work you can do is seemingly endless, and your concentration lasts for hours. I could happily stay in and read about the mechanics of Egyptian telecom systems or just as happily go out and chat to a mate. In Year 12 I wrote 16 pages for my TEE history exam in 50 minutes. When I only got 62 per cent, I was taken aback. I had included almost every fact I could remember about Stalin's rise to power and elaborated on all of them – that little bit too much, as my teacher informed me. The problem with dexies is that you get so excited about whatever it is you are talking or writing about, that you include information that may not be so riveting to others. Often more than once.

Some people, though, continue to use dexies throughout university and into their professional careers. Many of my friends at 26 still carry bottles of dexies on Friday nights out, just for that extra buzz. However, unless you are drunk, stoned or on any sort of 'calming' medication, the comedown from the dexies can be excruciating. Irritation and anxiety would take over from the high, leaving you feeling run-down, burnt out and empty.

Because of the amphetamine, we would often have to force down our first food for the day, be it a piece of fruit or bread, in a bid to get to sleep that night. The speed still circulating in your body long after the day is done makes getting to sleep difficult. We would always be prepared with a gram or so of bud (marijuana) or some downers such as diazepam, temazepam and the like that (as I can attest from personal experience) could be picked up from a local doctor by feigning a variety of symptoms. And of course heroin addicts themselves would always be 'doctor-shopping', re-enacting these scenes many times a day for different doctors and collecting piles of prescriptions, or simply stealing the pills from old people's homes, parents, medicine cabinets and hospitals...

For those of you who are still curious enough about the medication children have been taking, or have any doubts about whether it only 'works' on ADHD children, why don't you just go ahead and try them yourself? In my opinion, we should try what medication we give our kids in the way we once tested the temperature of the milk.

When I think of the strength of the drugs being given to children in this billion-dollar industry the rage I feel brings me to tears. Thanks to DSM-IV's list of subjective behavioural patterns, it is easy to get diagnosed with ADHD, and therefore be prescribed. Someone could claim to often make careless mistakes, often lose things, to dislike homework, often run late, often interrupt people, fail to do household chores and/ or confess to always being 'on the go'. It must be easy to convince doctors that one had a disorder when the list of symptoms could apply to almost anybody. At my school, kids would be prescribed bottles of 100 and sell them at school for between 20c and $1 per tablet. At exam times dexies would be in higher demand, as even people who usually refrained from taking them would like to have a few on stand-by for the long library hours. Some children were well aware of the sudden drought and increase in market and would up their prices to $1.50 or even $2 on the morning of the TEE exams. These kids weren't sick: they were budding little entrepreneurs.

When we'd take dexies for five days in a row, the sixth day was a nightmare. We would be fidgety, anxious, irritable and vague. When a 12-year-old girl at school was lowering her dosage she went through the same experience, sharing the same symptoms, as she was withdrawing. Someone mistook the symptoms of withdrawing for advanced ADHD and instead of continuing to lower her dosage, replaced it with a higher one. She went on to sell her medication at school, supposedly unbeknown to her parents.

The dexies were another form of currency within schools across the city. They could be traded for money, marijuana and so on. My best friend and I would buy 100 at a time to get us through the exam season. This was cheaper in the long run and ensured that we would have ample supply when the hordes came towards the end of the year.

Later, when we moved to Melbourne, we asked around for dexies and found that in comparison to WA, hardly anybody had any. When we looked into things a bit further we found that the diagnosis rate for ADHD in Perth was four times as high as it was elsewhere. We thought we might have to move back to Perth at first but managed to get on with our studies without them.

I stopped taking dexies at 17. But for many others who used dexies frequently at high school, this was just the beginning. Kids who had earlier turned up their noses at harder drugs, such as methamphetamine and heroin, had developed a love affair with getting high and were moving quickly to using bigger amounts of drugs. Methamphetamine became the weekend party drug for most late teenagers and kids in their early 20s.

The debate over whether they were self-medicating real illnesses, such as bipolar or ADHD, or whether they were just using drugs is still heated. But in my opinion the sheer amount of young adults using meth in the early 2000s in Perth was a great deal more than could ever possibly be 'sick'. Many Perth youths have lost friends to speed-induced psychosis, suicide and overdoses. Perth has a recreational drug problem. Dexies are not the cause of this, but they did play a large role in our appetite for highs in general while growing up.

I am 26 and teach children aged seven to ten. They don't like staying in their seats and they drive me up the wall. But when Darren throws a book at my head, call me conservative, but to administer him with psychotropic drugs isn't the first thing that comes to mind. I write this in response to the latest report to question the long-term benefit of stimulant medications in children. From experience, they have been far from beneficial to me. But the drugs still feel good and have very strong effects. And until we can make them feel bad, people will always abuse them.[28]

Holyoake: Working at the Coal Face

Like Clare Trevelyan, youth workers at Holyoake, a not-for-profit drug rehabilitation service based in Perth, are acutely aware of the reality of teenage amphetamine abuse. Mark Lowry, the former adolescent program co-ordinator at Holyoake, ran programs for fifteen- to eighteen-year-olds who were in trouble with the law and had been referred through the juvenile justice system. In 2004, 122 teenagers completed his program. He and other staff conducted interviews with new participants, asking them about their drug-taking habits. Sixty-nine (57 per cent) volunteered that they had abused dexamphetamine. Of those sixty-nine, only three were diagnosed with ADHD and abused their own dexamphetamine. Lowry thought that 57 per cent was an underestimate because participants knew dexamphetamine was a prescription drug and did not regard it as an illicit substance in the same way as they would cannabis or heroin. He estimated that the true figure would have been closer to 80 per cent.

Lowry identified common consequences of dexamphetamine abuse as being extreme mood swings, aggression, hyper-vigilance and paranoia. Another worrying consequence was hyper-sexuality, with teenagers prone to engage in unsafe sex, particularly when taking dexamphetamine while binge drinking.

Lowry believed that the mixed message about dexamphetamine being good for those who have ADHD but bad for those who do not, was not credible to teenagers. If it is good for the diagnosed children, and the federal government pays for it through the Pharmaceutical Benefits Scheme, it cannot be of any great harm. As a consequence they feel comfortable using dexamphetamine to manage their alcohol and, to a lesser extent, cannabis abuse. He believed that dexamphetamine normalised the amphetamine use and was a bridge to further drug abuse.[29]

Lessons Learned, Lessons Forgotten

While it took a long time, the lesson that amphetamine prescription facilitates amphetamine abuse was finally learned at the highest level in Western Australia. This was confirmed in September 2007 when the then premier Alan Carpenter told the Western Australian Parliament that 'the evidence shows that if amphetamine prescribing rates are decreased, abuse rates are decreased'.[30] It is a lesson, however, that has been learned and sometimes forgotten around the world many times before.

In 1968 Sweden withdrew Ritalin from the marketplace due to its escalating abuse. Swedish doctors and medical students felt 'considerable resentment' toward American medical journals that continued to advertise Ritalin. At the time Swedish doctors warned they saw 'no reason why similar abuse of central nervous system stimulants could not appear in other countries if their serious abuse potential is not carefully weighed against their rather limited therapeutic application'.[31] Thirty-seven years later, however, in June 2005, even Sweden forgot this lesson and the Swedish Medical Products Agency controversially took the decision to allow Ritalin back on the market. This was despite its history of abuse and the US FDA issuing warnings for potentially life-threatening psychiatric and cardiovascular risks.[32]

The potential for illicit diversion is recognised in laws enacted by all Australian states and territories making it illegal to possess, sell or use Schedule 8 drugs, including dexamphetamine and methylphenidate, without a medical prescription. Anyone found in possession of, or using, dexamphetamine without a prescription may be fined up to $2000 and/or receive a prison term of up to two years. Anyone convicted of selling or intent to sell dexamphetamine illegally may receive a fine of up to $100,000 and/or a prison term of up to twenty-five years.[33] Doctors providing the same addictive drugs in divertible quantities to children are rewarded.

More Detail Showing WA's History of High Amphetamine Abuse Rates

Interstate comparisons of dexamphetamine prescription rates and amphetamine abuse rates confirm that high prescribing rates are associated with high amphetamine abuse rates. In the 2003 Commonwealth Department of Health and Aged Care Survey the national rate of dexamphetamine prescriptions was 11.3 persons per 1000 population; Victoria reported the lowest rate of 6.7, while Western Australia was more than double the next highest state with a rate of 43.2.[34] In 2004 Western Australia had the highest level of amphetamine abuse of all states, with a rate of 4.5 per cent of the population aged fourteen years and over having abused amphetamines in the past year. This was well above the national average of 3.2 per cent. Victoria had one of the lowest rates of just 2.8 per cent.[35] The proportion of people presenting for treatment with amphetamine abuse as the principal drug of concern in 2005–06 also confirms this trend. The Australian average was 11 per cent of all treatment episodes with amphetamines identified as the principal drug of concern, while Western Australia reported the highest rate of 24.6 per cent and Victoria the lowest with a rate of 6.3 per cent.[36]

Other Risks

Addiction and abuse are not the only major risks associated with ADHD stimulants. Dexamphetamine has a vast range of potential adverse side effects. GlaxoSmithKline, the US manufacturers of Dexedrine (dexamphetamine) state the 'long-term effects of amphetamines in paediatric patients have not been well established' and list warnings for:

- sudden death at usual doses for ADHD for children and adults with pre-existing structural cardiac abnormalities or other serious heart problems;
- behaviour disturbance and thought disorder in patients with a pre-existing psychotic disorder;
- psychotic episodes, hallucinations, delusional thinking, or mania at usual doses in children and adolescents without a prior history of psychotic illness or mania;
- long-term suppression of growth;
- exacerbation of motor and phonic tics, and Tourette syndrome;
- aggressive behaviour or hostility, palpitations, tachycardia, elevation of blood pressure, over-stimulation, restlessness, dizziness, insomnia, euphoria, dyskinesia, dysphoria, tremor, headache, dryness of the mouth, unpleasant taste, diarrhoea, constipation, other gastrointestinal disturbances, anorexia, urticaria, impotence and other changes in libido.[37]

These are not abstract risks and they are not peculiar to dex-amphetamine. Ritalin, Concerta and Attenta all carry similar risks.[38] Some recent adverse events reported to the Australian Therapeutic Goods Administration (TGA) for Ritalin include: a seven-year-old boy who became 'depressed' and made a 'suicide attempt', and an eight-year-old boy who experienced 'hallucinations of spiders crawling on skin'.[39] At 19 March 2010 there had been 261 adverse event reports for stimulants. As reporting is voluntary there is no way of knowing what proportion of actual adverse events gets reported. A 2008 study by Curtin University pharmacologist Con Berbatis identified that only a tiny fraction (for general practitioners only 2 per cent) of adverse events are reported.[40] How many other children experienced hallucinations or attempted suicide will never be known.

Sample of Adverse Drug Reactions Committee (ADRAC) adverse event reports for Dexamphetamine and Methylphenidate

- boy (age unknown) who experienced 'growth retardation' and made a 'suicide attempt' (Ritalin);
- four-year-old boy who experienced 'seizures' and developed a 'rash' and 'blisters'. He also experienced 'diarrhoea, runny nose and coughing, and facial oedema' (Ritalin);
- Two eight-year-old boys who developed a 'psychotic disorder' (Ritalin);
- ten-year-old boy who began to do 'strange things and had full body tics and strange movements with his eyes' (Ritalin);
- thirteen-year-old boy who experienced a 'confusional state' and developed 'blurred vision, painful eyes, headaches, increased heart rate, swelling of face and lips, twitching and an increase in body temperature.' Patient also began hallucinating and felt that 'he had bugs on him', and he 'laughed for 10 minutes uncontrollably' (Ritalin);
- seventeen-year-old male patient a long-term user of dexamphetamine and Ritalin who 'attempted a sexual assault' after abusing alcohol and drugs. Possibility his original diagnosis was wrong in which case 'it was likely that his intellectual and psychological development had been severely affected' (dexamphetamine);

- seventeen-year-old girl who experienced 'aggression', 'violent behaviour' and 'uncontrollable sobbing and shakiness' (dexamphetamine).

Ritalin's Free Ride

Perhaps many of these adverse events could have been avoided had the TGA been more rigorous in assessing the safety and efficacy of Ritalin before approving it for use in Australia. In 1993 the TGA approved Ritalin for the treatment of ADHD despite advice from the Australian Drug Evaluation Committee (ADEC) that was highly critical of the data in relation to safety and adverse side effects.[41] ADEC commented:

> The data to support the use of methylphenidate in the treatment of ADHD have not been generated as a result of a co-ordinated, structured drug development program but rather in a somewhat haphazard manner by the various research groups in various locations over a long period of time. As a result the data package to support this application is deficient in certain areas when compared with that usually required by ADEC and the Department...The data on safety are the most deficient. No evaluable data on laboratory testing has been provided. Data on the incidence of adverse reactions was provided in only four of the short-term placebo-controlled trials. Long-term incidence data is confined only to the retrospective analysis of 250 children.[42]

Nine years later, in 2002, the TGA relied on similarly flawed information when it approved the heavier dosage drug Ritalin LA (long-acting). ADEC's comments on the submission supporting Ritalin LA included the following: 'The clinical evaluator draws attention to the increased risk of overdose posed by the Ritalin LA capsule compared with Ritalin immediate release tablets due to the increased strength of the LA formulation. There is also no safety data on Ritalin LA for longer than 12 weeks.'[43] In the absence of real data for Ritalin LA the TGA relied on the defective safety data from the original 1993 Ritalin application. The 'increased risk of overdose' for Ritalin LA over Ritalin should have required a rigorous safety analysis of Ritalin LA. Instead the mistakes of 1993 were repeated and compounded.

On 1 August 2005 the Commonwealth government subsidised Ritalin through the Pharmaceutical Benefits Scheme (PBS) for the treatment of ADHD. (See chapter 5.) This was despite the fact that a month earlier on 30 June 2005, the US Food and Drug Administration (FDA) issued a statement identifying serious safety concerns with methylphenidate.[44] (See chapter 4.) The TGA were aware of the emerging evidence in the month between the FDA's announcement and Ritalin being put on the PBS. In July 2005 a TGA spokeswoman told the *Australian Financial Review* that the TGA would 'monitor the deliberations of the FDA committee with interest' and that '[Australia's] Adverse Drug Reactions Advisory Committee has received 101 reports describing 238 adverse reactions in respect of methylphenidate since the product was first registered here'.[45] As soon as Ritalin was put on the PBS sales skyrocketed exposing thousands of children to these risks. Whether the TGA informed the Pharmaceutical Benefits Advisory Committee who recommended Ritalin for listing on the PBS is unclear, but it appears unlikely. (See appendix 1.)

The TGA's handling of Ritalin and Ritalin LA are not the only examples of its failure to protect Australian consumers. From January to September 2005 the FDA issued twenty black box warnings (see chapter 4) for drugs sold in both the US and Australia, while the Australian TGA issued warnings for only five of these twenty.[46] In response to a question on notice in the Senate, the TGA admitted that it didn't even bother to monitor the FDA's drug warnings.[47] In both countries the drugs are the same, the children are the same and the effects of drugs on patients are the same. Why bother even having a TGA if it is willing to accept defective foreign safety data to approve drugs, yet ignore emerging overseas evidence of the dangers of these drugs?

While most children don't experience extreme adverse reactions it is very common for children to experience insomnia, loss of appetite and/or personality changes. In 2001 a meta-analysis of sixty-two randomised trials with 2897 participants, was highly critical of pro-medication bias in publications and a lack of robustness in their findings, and found for methylphenidate products 'clinicians only need to treat 4 children to identify an episode of decreased appetite'.[48]

Despite this it is often claimed that the benefits of medicating for ADHD outweigh the risks. When asked for proof of the medications' effectiveness, 'experts' will often respond that there are thousands of scientific papers that support their claims. When asked, however, which one of these scientific papers has robust methodology, they cannot identify a single long-term research paper that withstands scrutiny.

Oregon ADHD Drug Effectiveness Review

Compelling evidence for the poor quality of this research was demonstrated in 2005 through the Oregon Health and Science University ADHD Drug Effectiveness Review Project. The review was commissioned by fifteen US states in order to determine which drugs were the safest and most cost effective.[49] The 731-page review analysed 2287 studies, 'virtually every investigation ever done on ADHD drugs anywhere in the world'.[50] Of the studies analysed, 'The group rejected 2,107 investigations as being unreliable, and reviewed the remaining 180 to find superior drugs'.[51] Instead of being able to make objective comparisons of the safety and effectiveness of the different drugs, the review was 'severely limited' by a lack of studies measuring 'functional or long-term outcomes'.[52]

The review concluded that 'evidence on the effectiveness of pharmacotherapy for ADHD in young children is seriously lacking'[53] and that there was 'no evidence on long-term safety of drugs used to treat ADHD in adolescents'.[54] The review also found that 'good quality evidence on the use of drugs to affect outcomes relating to global academic performance, consequences of risky behaviours, social achievements, etc. is lacking'.[55] It was also critical of the lack of research into the possibility that some ADHD drugs could stunt growth[56] and found that the evidence that ADHD drugs help adults was 'not compelling'.[57] Overall, the report ascertained that the body of evidence was of 'poor quality'.

I naively hoped the results of the Oregon Review would shake the foundation of the ADHD industry and bring a halt to the wholesale prescribing of amphetamines to children, but the findings were either ignored or dismissed with the mantra that the benefits of drugs 'clearly outweigh the risks'.[58]

Good science is not about quantity of research, it is about quality. None of the thousands of papers cited by ADHD proponents prove that ADHD is a biochemical imbalance or that amphetamines are safe and effective. Despite the 'paucity of evidence on the long term effects of psycho-stimulants on children'[59], parents are commonly reassured that stimulants have been used to control ADHD-like behaviour since the 1930s.[60] This begs the obvious question: why haven't the pharmaceutical companies set up a systematic review of the long-term effects of their products?

The MTA Study

Up until 2007 probably the most commonly referred to source justifying the use of drug therapy was the *Multimodal Treatment Study for Attention Deficit Hyperactivity Disorder* (aka the MTA Study). While there were several methodological flaws, notably a lack of a placebo and blind raters, the MTA Study did follow a significant number of children.[61] In 1999 after conducting the first fourteen months of the study the authors concluded that 'carefully crafted medication management was superior to the behavioural treatment and to routine clinical care that included medication'.[62] It was described as 'one of the first studies to demonstrate benefits of multimodal and pharmacological interventions lasting longer than 1 year' and became, I believe, the most frequently quoted single source supporting the use of stimulants for ADHD.[63]

However, in 2007, after an analysis of the three-year follow-up to the MTA Study, one of the scientists who ran the study, Professor William Pelham, concluded:

> I think we exaggerated the beneficial impact of medication in the first study. We had thought that children medicated longer would have better outcomes. That didn't happen to be the case...In the short run [medication] will help the child behave better, in the long run it won't. And that information should be made very clear to parents.[64]

The three-year data also showed that children using behavioural therapy alone had 'a slightly lower rate of substance abuse' and that 'the (medicated) children had a substantial decrease in their rate of growth, so they weren't growing as much as other kids in terms of both their height and their weight'.[65]

The fact that the fourteen-month data supported the use of stimulants and the three-year data did not, is also entirely in keeping with the commonsense proposition that children mature at different rates and 'that brains of children with ADHD, rather than developing abnormally (as in autism), mature later'.[66] It also supports the idea that while nothing affects behaviour as fast as behaviour-altering medications, amphetamines simply mask symptoms and do nothing to address their cause.

World's First Long-Term Data

The publication of the three-year data was a minor setback to the credibility of ADHD proponents, but it had no effect on Australian prescribing rates, which have skyrocketed since its publication. In reality, while the MTA Study hinted at sustained harm (stunted growth and drug abuse), it only followed children for three years, which is hardly long term. The data that showed significant evidence of long-term harm came from the Western Australian Ministerial Implementation Committee on ADHD (MICADHD, of which I was a member) Raine Study Review. The Review studied the data provided by the Raine Study, a long-term, large-scale, generalised study into children's health and wellbeing conducted at Perth's King Edward Memorial Hospital.[67] Published in February 2010 it provided the world's first independent data on the long-term effects (nine years) of psychostimulant medication.[68]

The two most significant findings of the MICADHD Raine Study Review were:

1. Long-term cardiovascular damage: 'The most noteworthy finding in the study was the association between stimulant medication and diastolic blood pressure. Compared to not receiving medication, the consistent use of stimulant medication was associated with a significantly higher diastolic blood pressure (of over 10mmHg). This effect did not appear to be solely attributable to any short-term effects of stimulant medication, as when comparing groups who were currently receiving medication, it was found that those who had consistently received medication at all time points had a significantly higher mean diastolic

blood pressure than those who had not consistently received medication in the past (difference of 7mmHg). These findings indicate there may be a lasting longer term effect of stimulant medication on diastolic blood pressure above and beyond the immediate short-term side effects.'[69]

2. School failure: 'In children with ADHD, ever receiving stimulant medication was found to increase the odds of being identified as performing below age-level by a classroom teacher by a factor of 10.5 times.'[70]

In addition the report indicated that there was a marginally negative outcome for both ADHD symptoms (inattention and hyperactivity) and depression with the long-term use of stimulant medication.[71]

The finding that amphetamine use may permanently raise diastolic blood pressure is of great significance. It had been previously recognised that while stimulants were in the patient's system, heart rate and blood pressure were elevated, leading to the associated risks of heart attacks and strokes. But it was assumed that when the short-term stimulant effects wore off the cardiovascular system returned to normal.

The most startling finding was that past stimulant use increased the probability of an ADHD child falling behind at school by a massive 950 per cent. This finding completely undermines the hypothetical basis of medicating for ADHD. As stated in the MICADHD report, the basis of the belief that amphetamines have long-term benefits are short-term studies, which 'indicate that immediate management of ADHD symptoms allows children to function more effectively within a classroom. It is hypothesised that this makes children more available for learning and allows children to learn skills and concepts which are necessary to function well within a classroom in the future.'[72] The analysis of the Raine Study data was the first time this hypothesis had been tested.

The suggestion that the Raine Study would be a possible source of long-term data on stimulant medication was first made by MICADHD members with a long history of prescribing and advocating the use of stimulants. They were obviously expecting very different results. I expected the results to show no long-term educational benefits or some adverse educational outcome from stimulants, but even I was surprised by the strength of the negative outcome. Initially, the medication proponents on MICADHD tried to claim that the outcomes for the medicated children were most probably worse than those for un-medicated children, because the medicated children had more severe ADHD. As a member of the committee, however, I insisted on a comparison of the groups at age five, which was prior to any of the children having been medicated. This analysis established that there were no statistically significant differences in developmental, behavioural and health measures before the children were medicated.

This did not prevent subsequent efforts to explain away this research using the unsupported hypothesis that differences in educational performance and the increase in blood pressure were due to pre-existing differences. Professor Ian Hickie from the Brain and Mind Research Institute dismissed the poor educational outcomes saying, 'typically those kids who go on the medication are considerably worse to start with'.[73] Hickie's comment needs to be seen in the light of his commercial ties to pharmaceutical companies. His CV acknowledges receipt of

$411,000 from four different pharmaceutical companies, mostly for research on psychotropic medications for depression, psychosis and bipolar disorder.[74] Even supposing Hickie's criticisms had been valid, and the children who had been medicated 'were considerably worse to start with', if amphetamines worked, they should have been performing at least as well at school as those with moderate, un-medicated ADHD.

As with all studies there are limitations with the MICADHD study. While the sample size (131) was small, 'it was larger than those in many short-term studies that supported the use of stimulants as a safe and effective treatment for children with ADHD'.[75] Although the evidence now available from the Review does not prove beyond all doubt that amphetamines cause failure at school and permanent cardiovascular damage, it is compelling. When this evidence was published I called for the removal of ADHD stimulants from the PBS in the full knowledge that because of vested interests, and 'inertia', it would not happen. If childhood psychiatric practice was 'evidence-based' and precautionary, the evidence should have immediately halted the explosion in national child prescription rates, but of course it did not. There was too much money and too many professional reputations at stake.

The legal implications of this research, however, have the capacity to fundamentally change medical practice. Nothing scares incompetent doctors, or more importantly their insurers, more than competent lawyers. Since it was published in February 2010, doctors prescribing ADHD stimulants to children have been accepting legal liability for potential educational or cardiovascular damage. Perhaps the legal profession will succeed where the medical profession has failed.

3

True Believers

ADHD is a catch-all diagnosis, with the promise of a magic bullet treatment that suits financially wealthy, but time-poor, societies. Prescribing rates have exploded because it is in the interests of many stakeholders to accept, without proof, the hypothesis that ADHD is caused by a biochemical imbalance. Drug companies profit, busy clinicians get a quick, easy, lucrative diagnosis and treatment, struggling teachers get a compliant child, governments get a cheap way of appearing to meet child mental health demands and parents are fooled into an illusory belief that they have helped their child with a quick and apparently effective intervention. The real losers in the ADHD debate are children who are completely powerless to prevent themselves being 'medicated'.

Parents

Parents usually dread hearing that their child has a disease or disorder, especially when they are told that it is incurable and possibly lifelong.[1] Yet paradoxically many parents welcome, and actively seek, a diagnosis of ADHD for their child. Some even seek a second opinion if the original doctor won't confirm their strongly held belief that their child has ADHD and needs medicating. Often parents are relieved when they are told that their child's real or perceived behavioural problems are not a result of their parenting. Many loving but ill-informed parents are convinced that they must 'medicate' their child to ensure they don't suffer the 'debilitating fate' of undiagnosed and un-medicated ADHD sufferers. Some look back at their own lives and attribute educational, social, career and relationship difficulties to their own undiagnosed ADHD. (See chapter 1.)

Sometimes parents feel apprehensive and a little guilty about their decision to medicate their child, and it is only human to look for evidence that validates important decisions. The fact that a child is more focused and obedient after taking medication reassures parents that they have made the right decision. Other parents, however, become concerned about the loss of spontaneity and creativity in their child.

Whatever the attitude of parents, the reality is that in allowing their children to be chemically altered they risk a host of side effects, risks that parents often remain uninformed about. (See chapter 2.) And sometimes parents, fully aware of these risks, are seduced into believing their child is 'chemically unbalanced' without amphetamines in their system and persist with the use of stimulants.

Parenting is difficult. The interaction between challenging behaviours and family dysfunction is complex, with each potentially causing the other. Effective parents help children to learn and to behave in socially acceptable ways. It is an unpleasant yet obvious reality that some ill-equipped parents will cause ADHD-type behaviours in their children no matter how well meaning they may be. These parents not only cause the behaviours, but are also the primary source of the behavioural 'evidence' used for the diagnosis.

ADHD proponents simplify this difficult equation by removing responsibility from parents. Peter Breggin believes their message to parents is: 'You are not the cause and you are not the cure...We are doctors; we have the knowledge and we have the treatments.'[2] Naturally many parents often take doctors' advice at face value and allow their children to be medicated – their child's changed behaviour confirmation of the ADHD diagnosis. This has been the experience of the Perth-based Bentley Health Service ADHD team whose submission to the 2004 Western Australian Parliamentary Inquiry into ADHD (see chapter 6) stated:

> We have observed that once medication has been commenced, it is often difficult to convince the family to consider reducing or ceasing the medication as it has created the 'perfect child'...a child who has become frozen – in effect quietened and serious in nature, certainly not your typical child.[3]

Professor of Psychology, Paediatrics and Psychiatry and the director of the Research Unit on Children's Psycho-Social

Maladjustment at the University of Montreal, Richard Tremblay questions the very concept of the 'functional child':

> Children are born antisocial, they don't become anti-social. They don't know the rules of society, things like compromising and taking turns, unless we teach them. That's why we see temper tantrums and lots of misbehaviour in very young children.[4]

According to Tremblay, children, particularly boys, need 'to learn the rules of society'.[5] A failure to learn the rules is a logical consequence of not having been taught these behaviours. The notion said above that a child diagnosed with ADHD is biologically impaired assumes that normal impulse control happens in a vacuum. It assumes maturity is a consequence of age rather than experience. It assumes good manners are biologically determined and not learned.

The way parents interact with their child obviously influences the child's behaviour. Commonsense considerations, however, can be swamped by the professional credibility of a doctor who tells a parent their child, and possibly they, have a genetically predetermined biochemical brain imbalance that's treatable with medication. It is also much easier for a clinician to suggest a biological problem than to ask parents to confront their own inadequacies. It is a brave clinician who will suggest to parents that the family dynamic may be the problem. An ADHD diagnosis helps some parents avoid that unpleasant reality and saves the clinician from having to ask difficult and confronting questions.

Typical of this absolution from parental responsibility is the following statement by Perth paediatrician, now retired from ADHD prescribing, Dr Ken Whiting:

> The concept of a 'dysfunctional family' should be approached with care and has been over-diagnosed in the past – as ADHD is an inherited disorder, it is highly likely that one or more adults in the family will also have attention deficit/hyperactivity disorder.[6]

On the advice of 'experts' like Dr Whiting, some parents are convinced that their child has inherited ADHD from them, and are also diagnosed and medicated. This is the genius of ADHD marketing. Parents whose children are 'medicated' can become customers, and even spokespeople for the ADHD industry, happy to share their success stories about ADHD medication. These stories, told by parents grateful for the chemically enhanced improvements in themselves and their child, are then used to market the condition, the drugs and the ADHD specialists, through favourable media coverage.

The following excerpt from Perth's *Sunday Times* is an example of this tactic (although the article itself was contained within a balanced feature titled 'Drugging Our Young', which fairly presented the different perspectives on ADHD):

> Giving psychotropic drugs to her child is not an agonising choice for Kathy [name changed]. On the contrary, she is relieved. Relief that a medical reason explained her son's behaviour, relief that science found a product to manage the symptoms, relief he has an education...Without stimulants, odds are that

Andrew [name changed] would have been expelled from school, probably with few friends and fewer job prospects. Now 15, Andrew has been taking dexamphetamines or Ritalin since he was a seven-year-old. 'I'm not normal,' he explains. 'If I was to sit down and jot a graph for you of taking pills, it would go up and gradually go down and then, crash. If I forget my pills, I'm off my nut'...Kathy says Andrew's Year 2 teacher filled out a questionnaire and suggested she take it to the doctor.

She saw one of Perth's prominent behavioural paediatricians, Trevor Parry, who diagnosed ADHD (inattentive-type) after two sessions – one with her and Andrew, one with Andrew alone. There were no whole-family sessions and she recalls no referrals to a psychiatrist or other counsellors. 'It was miraculous,' she says. 'The first day, I gave him his little pill in the morning and then went to class that afternoon to pick him up and he had stickers and a certificate. The teacher and I were both so pleased; we were beaming from ear to ear.'

Kathy hopes that once school and TAFE are over, he will be mature enough to stop the pills. 'It's all about school, really,' she says. 'He only has one chance at an education. At least when he's medicated, he does have some focus.'[7]

Kathy and Andrew's story contains many of the typical elements of an ADHD success story:
- parents' relief that 'medical' reasons explained their child's behaviour;

- fear of the consequences of not medicating – being expelled from school, having few friends and few prospects;
- damage to the child's self-perception: 'I'm not normal';
- ignorance by the child and presumably the parent of the withdrawal effects of amphetamines: 'If I forget my pills, I'm off my nut';
- an enthusiastic teacher who first suggested the diagnosis and provided the supporting evidence (and may have suggested an appropriate doctor);
- the teachers' and the parents' suspicions confirmed by the ADHD-specialising paediatrician, without reference to a second opinion or a trial of non-drug alternatives;
- the 'miraculous' and immediate 'first day' behavioural change delivered by stimulants;
- the pleasure of both parent and 'beaming' teacher that the problem child is no longer a problem;
- the parents' angst about educational prospects with 'only one chance at an education';
- the hope that the child will become mature enough to stop the pills despite the perception by the child he is 'not normal' and without medication he is 'off his nut'.

Andrew may well have been 'off his nut' when he came off his medication, but not necessarily because he had some underlying medical problem. His being 'off his nut' is typical of the withdrawal or 'rebound' effects of stimulants. (See chapter 2.)

Julian James, a former clinical nurse specialist at Western Australia's Community Child and Adolescent Mental Health Clinic – Bentley Health Service, believes the rebound effect is not just biochemical but also psychological: 'The child is unfamiliar with how to respond because they don't have the chemicals on board and we often find they are frustrated. They can be violent and it takes a while before that settles down. And then we're able to start working with them.'[8] The majority of the children seen by the Bentley ADHD team diagnosed with the disorder leave diagnosis and medication free.[9] In 2006 Dr Helen Milroy, a former psychiatrist at the clinic, said, 'we need to be clear what we are talking about in regards to medication, we are not saying we are teaching children how to manage without medication, we are not medicating them because they don't require it for the diagnosis we have given them'.[10]

The Bentley ADHD team is rare in that the staff work with parents as well as children and, where necessary, challenge parents to confront how their own behaviour is affecting their child. The team demand much of parents and there are many inspiring success stories from Bentley; however, some parents are unable to sustain the necessary changes and revert to old habits, including medicating their child.

One notable success story is that of Brandon Frances and his mother Katherine, who sustained the difficult permanent changes initiated by the Bentley ADHD team. Brandon was first medicated for behavioural problems when he was four. By early 2004, Brandon (then twelve) was on dexamphetamine for ADHD, sodium valproate for mood stabilisation and tranquillisers to calm him down. As a result of this toxic cocktail Brandon suffered mood swings, migraines and insomnia. He sleepwalked, had chronic stomach aches and was unnaturally thin. The Bentley team provided Brandon with a residential intensive intervention program which turned around his life and that of his family. He was initially detoxified, and his mother Katherine participated in effective parenting sessions. Brandon's hearing and learning difficulties were correctly identified as his real problems and he is now drug-free, and a happy and responsible young man.

Support Groups

Having made the emotional decision to 'medicate' their child and perceiving an improvement in their child's behaviour, some parents are keen to share their life-changing experience with others. They become active in parent support groups like Children and Adults with Attention Deficit Hyperactivity Disorder (CHADD) in the USA and the Learning and Attentional Disorders Society (LADS) in Perth, Western Australia.

Like most patient support groups both CHADD and LADS receive funds from the pharmaceutical industry.[11] Investigative health journalist Ray Moynihan believes the drug companies sponsor these support groups as a means of 'helping to paint a picture of an under-diagnosed medical disorder best treated with drugs'.[12] These groups, however, are not puppets of the drug companies. Rather, CHADD or LADS and the drug companies are partners with identical positions on ADHD. Only their motivations differ: the pharmaceutical companies seek profits and share price increases; the support groups are convinced they are helping children and families.

In 1998 when I was a teacher curious and concerned about ADHD, I attended a LADS forum in a packed hall in South Perth. Although I am not and never have been religious, and therefore have a limited frame of reference, it seemed to me more like a church service than a science-based information forum. Participants talked about their life-transforming experiences once they or their child had been diagnosed and medicated. Presenters invited those in the audience who were having difficulty getting diagnosed to visit clinicians who embraced the condition. I was disappointed with what I perceived as a lack of balance and was concerned about the evangelical feel of the event.

I have no doubt the majority of active members of LADS are motivated by their fervent belief in ADHD and in the wonderful life-changing benefits of medication. Similarly, Moynihan considers that CHADD is no mere 'advocacy group' but more like a 'highly energised political or religious organisation'.[13] In 2003 CHADD chief executive officer E. Clark Ross admitted that the 'science' to support the validity of ADHD 'really is a matter of belief'.[14] Where LADS and CHADD differ from the churches and other faith-based organisations is in their advocacy of prescribing amphetamines to children.

As absurd as it sounds, CHADD honours high-profile ADHD ideologues in the 'ADHD Hall of Fame'. Inductees include Distinguished Professor of Psychiatry at the University of Utah School of Medicine, Paul Wender.[15] In 1995 Wender claimed to have found the holy grail of the ADHD movement, a reliable biological marker, foot tapping! According to Wender:

Fidgeting and foot movements (known in our research setting as 'Wender's sign') are very common signs of hyperactivity in adult ADHD patients – so much so that such patients can usually be diagnosed in the waiting room by a knowledgeable receptionist...I seriously entertain the possibility that this foot movement may be a biological marker for ADHD[16]...[T]he reduction of the foot sign in ADHD patients may also be an indicator of stimulant [drug] response.[17]

That Wender is held in high enough regard by CHADD to be inducted into the ADHD Hall of Fame speaks volumes about the credibility of both.

LADS

CHADD has been enormously influential in the US where drug companies can advertise directly to consumers. However, in Australia this is not the case, which makes pharmaceutical companies potentially more reliant on ADHD support groups to help them maximise patient numbers and profits. Like CHADD, LADS is partially funded by drug companies and has a long history of marketing the stock-standard line of ADHD as having a biological cause best treated with 'safe', 'effective' medication.[18]

LADS also frequently reassures parents they are not a cause of their child's behaviour. A LADS ADHD fact sheet produced by Perth Clinical Psychologist Derek Cohen begins:

If I had to select one fundamental issue to comment on in the therapy of ADHD children it would be the erroneous conclusion drawn by many parents and professionals alike that ADHD children have behaviour problems that simply require more discipline. While ADHD children present with problem behaviours, these are due to underlying neuropsychological factors.[19]

In a 2004 paid community newspaper advertisement for LADS, executive officer Michelle Toner was quoted as saying:

> [ADHD was] caused by an imbalance of the chemical dopamine in the brain…it was as inheritable as height and could create problems with inattention, impulsiveness, memory, organisation, time management and hyperactivity…not all people diagnosed with ADHD were hyperactive and the extreme behaviours often associated with it were uncharacteristic…ADHD medication had been used since 1937 and the 'hysteria' sometimes associated with it was often unfounded and uninformed.[20]

These statements of hypothesis as fact are typical of the information provided by LADS and were relatively moderate by their standards. In 2003, on a Perth community television program *Face the Facts*, speaking on behalf of LADS, Michelle Toner and psychiatrist Dr Roger Patterson made some noteworthy statements. Dr Patterson said:

> dexamphetamine has the amphetamine name in it and this is what people are starting to worry about because they are giving them to children – or they are taking them themselves…let me dispel that, they are taking a medicinal form of amphetamine…this is not addictive stuff. In fact, I wish it was a little more addictive so that my younger patients would remember to take it rather than having to be reminded by their long-suffering parents.[21]

Toner's statements on the same TV program were even more notable. 'In order to get a high equivalent to what people are taking [as] street speed, you would have to take close to 200 tablets. Children take 1 or 6 tablets a day and it is not addictive at all.'[22] Two hundred of the standard 5 milligram dexamphetamine tablets would deliver a dose of 1 gram which would kill most people and a fair proportion of elephants as well.[23]

Also obviously ignorant of the effects of 1 gram of dexamphetamine, the interviewer went on to ask Toner: 'Right, but if you do have ADHD and you take the medication, is it successful?' Toner replied, 'Oh yes...a lot of people discovered they had ADHD by accident. For example, truckies who needed uppers to keep them awake while they were driving across the Nullarbor suddenly found that they were driving a whole lot better...when they were taking dexies.'[24] As for Michelle Toner's claim about truckies driving a 'a whole lot better', she was presumably unaware that driving with non-prescription dexamphetamine is illegal and carries penalties including disqualification from driving, fines and/or imprisonment. Research has found that rather than 'driving a whole lot better' people who use dexamphetamine illicitly or for ADHD make more mistakes while driving, probably because the drug causes tunnel vision which stops them seeing peripheral information like red lights.[25]

In the 1990s LADS was unrestrained in its enthusiasm for the use of psychostimulants. The group was even warned twice not to recommend the illegal use of a child's stimulant by parents. Minutes from meetings of the Western Australian Stimulants Committee (formed to monitor the prescription of psychostimulants, see chapter 5) revealed that in August 1998 the Committee wrote to LADS asking it to stop advising parents to take their child's medication if they thought they had adult ADHD.[26]

As the ADHD debate in Perth evolved and concerns about over-diagnosis and over-prescription gained media coverage, LADS became a little more subtle, but never wavered in its support for the use of medication as the first line treatment. Instead of completely dismissing alternative treatments they began to talk about multimodal treatment. In my experience, multimodal treatment as LADS terms it means medication first, supported by other secondary treatments. While their language may have moderated a little, the line between LADS and the drug companies remains blurred.

I believe that the members of LADS are well intentioned, and that LADS provides some useful support to parents, such as information about strategies for helping inattentive students with their homework. Nevertheless, this good work is overshadowed by both its unquestioning and emotional promotion of ADHD medications and its financial ties to the pharmaceutical companies.

In the following press release, prepared by public relations business Last Say Communications, LADS provides the human face for Concerta, thus creating an emotionally charged sense of urgency about the need for this long-acting form of methylphenidate:

ADHD: A Day of Calm – Dawn to Dusk Long Lasting Medication to Provide Relief for Kids with ADHD

From April 1st 2007, an effective way of delivering medication over a 12-hour period will be available on the PBS and help children with ADHD normalise their lives. This long acting form of methylphenidate (Concerta) will overcome the stigma of taking their daily medication during school hours, an issue faced by many children with ADHD.

'School can be hell for kids with ADHD,' says Michelle Toner of the Learning and Attentional Disorders Society (LADS), an organisation supporting children with Attention Deficit Hyperactivity Disorder (ADHD) and their parents.

'We always have a box of tissues handy at the LADS office for mums who drop their kids off at school and then come in for a cry.

'Often, the worst problem faced by these kids is the attitude of other children, and the stigma of carrying the ADHD label. Parents work long and hard with teachers to put strategies in place which help their children cope with the demands of the classroom and playground.

'Medication is often a valuable part of their treatment plan, but the vast majority can only afford short-acting versions, which require a lunchtime dose to be taken at school.'

'Young people hate being singled out like that, and many schools don't like the responsibility of medicating children. As a result lots of kids refuse to take their lunchtime dose. For them schoolwork becomes harder, the playground becomes a minefield, and bullying often occurs.

'The inclusion of a sustained release methylphenidate on the PBS will be welcomed by these families. Not only will it assist with the school day, but tackling homework should become a lot easier as well'.[27]

Pharmaceutical companies sponsor research that they believe will paint a favourable picture of their products and have the ability to suppress the publication of unfavourable results. They must, however, at least pay lip service to the scientific process and are limited by law from making claims about their products that are completely false. Because CHADD and LADS are separate and independent entities from drug companies, when support groups exaggerate the benefits and deny the risks of medications, they increase drug company sales and profits without exposing the drug companies to any legal liability.

Teachers and Schools

Although teachers do not diagnose children with ADHD, they, along with parents, provide the critical evidence for the doctors who make the diagnosis. In 2003 US research demonstrated 'that in the majority of cases teachers are the first to suggest a diagnosis of ADHD'.[28] This is also common in Australia. Even if teachers are not the first to suggest a diagnosis they still play a central role in the process. If a teacher has to complete an ADHD checklist on little Johnny's behaviour and he has had a bad week and been misbehaving, it is natural that this will influence how the teacher reports his behaviour. At least parents usually attend the appointment with the diagnosing clinician, but information from teachers is most often limited to tick-box questionnaires and they often have no capacity to explain or qualify their responses. Some may be completely unaware of their role in the diagnostic process, and completely ignorant that their tick-box response that little Johnny often (rather than sometimes) is disorganised or distracted could mean the difference between him not meeting the diagnostic threshold or being diagnosed ADHD and put on amphetamines.

Some teachers prefer quiet, ordered classrooms. Others have a more laissez-faire approach. What a strict teacher perceives as 'butting in' another may perceive as participating in classroom discussion. DSM-IV states that children may not display ADHD behaviours if they are in an 'especially interesting activity or situation'.[29] Therefore if a child has a teacher who interests them, they will display ADHD behaviours less often. Conversely, boring teachers bore students, who then fidget, lose focus and misbehave. Similarly, incompetent teachers who lack the skills to effectively engage a class will, as a result of their incompetence, create inattentive and disruptive behaviour in students. These boring or incompetent teachers then provide the observational evidence that is used to diagnose ADHD.

In 2004 Perth Montessori school principal Gary Pears said 'political correctness' is hampering proper treatment of the issue: 'It [ADHD] does have a lot to do with parenting. It also has to do with teaching. Young, newly graduated, female teachers want these boys to sit down, shut up. It's about recognising difference and tolerating individuality.'[30] When interviewed in February 2008 the then Member of the Western Australian Parliament and former school teacher, the late Paul Andrews MLA, said:

I worked in a school which employed first-year female teachers, the vast majority of whom could not control classes of fourteen- and fifteen-year-old, normal, boisterous boys. They often referred these boys to the school psychologist who was a firm believer in ADHD.

These teachers referred increasing numbers because it got the boys out of class and made the classes easier to control. As a consequence the number of referrals increased rapidly as did the number of boys diagnosed with ADHD. When these students were in other classes with experienced teachers, they were not a problem.[31]

ADHD-type behaviours can be disruptive in a classroom and, as we have seen, children can be more compliant when medicated. Often teachers provide glowing reports to parents about how their newly medicated child is more attentive and focused in class. This is frequently cited as evidence of improved academic performance when it simply reflects the fact that the child is easier to control. I think I was a good teacher with effective classroom management techniques, and the boys I taught were on the whole attentive, motivated and easy to control. Even I had days when boisterous annoying behaviour, by a few, made the job of educating the many more difficult.

When difficult children are medicated, other students may benefit from a quieter learning environment and more of the teacher's time. Children displaying ADHD-type behaviours, however, do not represent a danger to others. For whose benefit are we drugging the ADHD child? If some children's behaviour prevents other class members from learning then it may be appropriate to remove the disruptive child from the classroom. But there is absolutely no justification for medicating children to keep them quiet in order to improve the learning outcomes of others.

Philosophies of inclusion, if they are to be more than merely words, must mean that children are included as they are and not made compliant via pharmaceutical interventions. The educational practices of previous generations, such as corporal punishment, are today regarded as barbaric. As adults, how will today's children view the widespread medicating of their generation? Will they view their parents' generation, which allowed drugging for compliance, more or less favourably than their grandparents' generation which allowed caning?

The diagnostic criteria of ADHD − in particular making careless mistakes, not 'seeming to' listen, failing to finish school work, being disorganised, disliking schoolwork or homework, blurting out answers and leaving a seat when remaining seated is expected − are all evidence of a child's failure to comply in a school environment. But which is the problem, the child or the environment? Despite the rhetoric of student-focused education, the vast majority of classrooms still operate in the traditional manner, where the teacher sets common tasks and students of varying ability and disposition are expected to complete them. The emphasis on mainstreaming an increasingly diverse range of students with a one-size-fits-all approach means there are an increasing number of 'square peg' students in 'round hole' classrooms.

A diagnosis of ADHD removes responsibility from the school and shifts 'the focus away from what might be wrong with schooling to centre only on what is "wrong" with the child'.[32] The environment is not modified to fit the child; instead the child is modified (medicated) to fit the environment. These are not new concerns. In 1970, in response to the emerging practice of drugging for hyperactivity, American author and educator John Holt, testifying about the US education system before a House of Representatives committee said:

We consider it [hyperactivity] a disease because it makes it difficult to run our schools as we do, like maximum security prisons, for the comfort and the convenience of the teachers and administrators who work in them. The energy of children is 'bad' because it is a nuisance to the exhausted and overburdened adults who do not want to or know how to and are not able to keep up with it. Given the fact that some children are more energetic and active than others, might it not be easier, more healthy, and more humane to deal with this fact by giving them more time and scope to make use of and work off their energy?…Everyone is taken care of, except, of course, the child himself, who wears a label which to him reads clearly enough 'freak,' and who is denied from those closest to him, however much sympathy he may get, what he and all children most need – respect, faith, hope, and trust.[33]

These comments are as relevant in Australia today as they were in America when they were made. Far from including students with challenging behaviours defined as ADHD, many Australian schools have threatened their exclusion unless their parents agree to have them medicated. In January 2007, the Brisbane *Courier Mail* reported that students refusing to medicate were excluded from Queensland schools, even although it was illegal to do so. It reported the case of Denise, a northside Brisbane mother and her son John, who had been branded a 'bad' child all through pre-school. 'This came to a head when he had only been in Grade 1 for approximately four months when the principal came to me and told me I either put my son on medication or he would be expelled.'[34] Linda Graham, a Queensland University of Technology PhD student who had just completed a related study, backed up the claims stating, 'Parents of children who can be described as "hyperactive" or "distractable" are under pressure to medicate their children so they can fit into an overwrought, under-funded public education system.'[35]

This is not limited to Queensland. In 2006, a public primary school located in a disadvantaged area of Sydney made headlines by threatening to formally exclude an eight-year-old girl unless her mother medicate her for suspected ADHD.[36] I know similar exclusions have occurred in Western Australia. A truly inclusive education system would recognise and cater for difference. Philosophies of inclusion must be supported with the resources needed to cater for individual needs.

The practice of excluding un-medicated ADHD children from schools became so common in the US that some states took action to protect children and their parents from state-enforced medicating. In 1999, Colorado legislated to prevent school personnel from recommending psychotropic drugs to students, with other states following. The legislation does not stop teachers and other school employees, however, recommending to parents that their child should be assessed by a doctor.[37]

Doctors

Ultimately the explosion in ADHD prescribing rates is primarily the result of bad doctoring rather than bad parenting or teaching. While some parents actively seek a diagnosis of ADHD for their child, the majority of parents are like their children, passive victims, who take professional advice at face value. These parents should not feel guilty if that advice is wrong. They are not the ones who prescribed the medication. Responsibility for prescribing dangerous drugs to modify the behaviour of children rests with the doctor. The readiness of some clinicians to prescribe is in part due to the fact that alternatives demand more time, money and emotional investment. Rather than tell parents they can't help their child, many clinicians feel obligated to do something. This is no excuse for subjecting children to potential adverse effects and abandoning their Hippocratic oath to 'first do no harm'.

In April 2006 the Western Australian magazine *Medical.WA Forum* conducted a poll of 245 Western Australian general practitioners. Three and a half times as many GPs thought ADHD drugs were over-prescribed as those who thought they were not.[38] While the majority clearly have concerns about prescribing rates, they are, with a few notable exceptions, a silent majority who abandon the field and don't participate in the public debate.[39] They allow a minority of ADHD proponents, typically heavy prescribers, to dominate the debate and make ADHD a mainstream disorder.

In contrast to sceptical doctors, frequent prescribers often have a lot invested in the validity of ADHD. Diagnosis and prescribing, or research, is a major proportion of their income, and they have invested professional credibility and their public profile. Some even have their family members 'medicated' for the condition. Effectively this enthusiastic minority have come to dominate mainstream paediatric medical practice.

4

Uncle Sam Knows Best

The Australian drug safety regulator, the Therapeutic Goods Administration (TGA), is heavily reliant on the US Food and Drug Administration (FDA), which means that Australian consumers are too. That does not mean to say that the FDA regulates well. Recent revelations from whistleblowers within the FDA have revealed a history of improper drug company influence on decisions and processes. Additionally, the reliance of Australian medical practice, particularly psychiatry, on imported American Psychiatric Association diagnostic criteria, over which the Australian medical profession has no control, leaves Australian consumers doubly vulnerable.

Chapter five of the *International Clarification of Diseases* 10 (ICD-10) is the criterion for mental health disorders published by the World Health Organization and used predominantly in Europe. It is largely overlooked in Australia. The eighteen diagnostic criteria for hyperkinetic disorder outlined in ICD-10 are virtually identical to those for ADHD in the *Diagnostic and Statistical Manual of Mental Disorders* (DSM-IV). There are, however, two subtle but important distinctions. First, for a diagnosis of hyperkinetic disorder, an individual is required to display at least six of nine of the inattentive *and* three of five of the hyperactive *and* one of four of the impulsive behaviours. For a DSM-IV diagnosis of ADHD, six of nine of the inattentive *or* six of nine of the hyperactive/impulsive are sufficient. Second, unlike ADHD, hyperkinetic disorder is not diagnosed if another condition that may explain the behaviour is diagnosed.

While many of the criticisms of subjectivity of assessment of behaviours are common to both the DSM-IV and ICD-10, in practice far fewer children are diagnosed using ICD-10. Despite the fact that Australia is a member of the World Health Organization and obviously not the American Psychiatric Association, DSM-IV is the predominant criteria used in Australia. As a consequence, the rate of psychostimulant use per head in the US and Western Australia (using DSM-IV) between 1994 and 2000 was approximately ten times the UK rate (predominantly using ICD-10).[1]

This is not only true for ADHD, DSM-IV generally contains looser, less rigorous diagnostic criteria than ICD-10. A 2005 study compared diagnosis rates for a range of childhood psychiatric disorders using the diagnostic criteria in DSM-IV and the equivalent disorder in ICD-10. For the majority of disorders, including ADHD, rates of diagnosis were higher using DSM-IV.[2] Rather than seeing this as a strength of ICD-10, the authors of the study saw this as a weakness. They suggested that using ICD-10 could lead to a failure to treat appropriately an 'ill-defined category which may include very different conditions such as excessive masturbation and thumb-sucking'.[3] They failed to specify what constituted excessive thumb sucking and masturbation and what constituted appropriate levels. Their strange concerns aside, a legitimate question remains: why is DSM-IV and not ICD-10 the dominant criterion used in Australia?

The American Psychiatric Association

The American Psychiatric Association has a long history of pathologising as disorders behaviours they consider 'abnormal' or 'immoral'. In 1952 the original *Diagnostic and Statistical Manual of Mental Disorders* (DSM-I) classified homosexuality as a 'sexual deviation disorder', as did DSM-II in 1968. In December 1973 DSM-II was modified by the Board of Trustees of the APA. The Board voted to eliminate the general category of homosexuality, and replace it with 'sexual orientation disturbance'.

The removal of homosexuality as a disorder went against the long-term trend of ever increasing numbers of disorders being added. The first 1952 edition was 130 pages long and contained 106 disorders. The latest edition published in 2000, DSM-IVTR, contains 943 pages and 297 disorders. One of the more bizarre disorders the manual currently recognises is 'mathematics disorder', where an individual is poor at maths relative to other subjects.[4] Instead of being regarded as poor at maths and good at English, students with relatively poor maths skills are now disordered. Fortunately no pharmaceutical interventions have as yet been identified.

Partly in response to increasing competition from non-medical mental health practitioners, psychiatry has increasingly become dominated by the 'pill for every ill' medical model. Psychologists, counsellors and social workers are all able to offer professional talking therapies as alternatives to psychiatry. Even friends and family can offer informal chats and advice. The licence to medically intervene either pharmacologically or through surgery is psychiatry's major marketing edge.

Prominent anti-ADHD campaigner Dr Peter Breggin believes market forces are the motivation for the cosy relationship between the APA and pharmaceutical companies:

> In the 1970s, the APA was going broke. Many psychiatrists were having difficulty filling their practices. Always near the bottom of the medical income scale, psychiatrists were floundering economically. Competition from non-medical professionals was cutting heavily into private practices...In the early 1980s, the APA made a decision that changed its history and that of our society. It decided to create an economic and political partnership with the drug companies. The partnership would enable psychiatry to use drug company funds to promote the medical model, psychopharmacology, and the authority and influence of psychiatry. Backed by the multi-billion dollar drug industry, psychiatry hoped to defeat the threat from non-medical professionals, such as psychologists and social workers. Within a scant few years, APA transformed itself from a failing institution into one of the most powerful political forces in the nation. It developed lobbying groups in state

capitals and in Washington, DC; gained a stronger influence in the media and the courts; and distributed increasing numbers of drugs to escalating numbers of people. Psychiatry's decision to save itself by going into partnership with the drug companies was an openly discussed survival plan.[5]

Even within the American Psychiatric Association questions have long been asked about the appropriateness of their relationship with the pharmaceutical industry. In 1985 Fred Gottlieb, APA Speaker of the House, told the APA:

> I do not suggest that either they [the drug companies] or we [the American Psychiatric Association] are evil folks. But I continue to believe that accepting such money is, in the long run, inimical to our independent functioning. We have evolved a somewhat casual and quite cordial relationship with the drug houses, taking their money readily...We seem to discount available data that drug advertising promotes irrational prescribing practices. We seem to think that we as psychiatrists are immune from the kinds of unconscious emotional bias in favour of those who are overtly friendly toward us...We persist in ignoring an inherent conflict of interest.[6]

To restore its credibility as an organisation concerned with science, and with patient welfare, the APA must change emphasis from hypothesising new disorders and managing symptoms to finding causes and cures. Too many psychiatric disorders have been hypothesised as being caused by, and subsequently treated as, a biochemical imbalance. In 2000, Harvard University Medical School psychiatrist and author Joseph Glenmullen stated: 'In every instance where such an imbalance was thought to have been found, it was later proven false.'[7] American psychiatry has a horrid history of getting it wrong. Psychiatry has, unlike every other medical discipline, been spectacularly unsuccessful at finding cures. Dr Harold Pincus, vice chairman of the *Diagnostic and Statistical Manual of Mental Disorders* task force was quoted in 2000 as saying, 'There has never been any criterion that psychiatric diagnoses require a demonstrated biological aetiology.'[8] Clearly the APA thinks that it is not crucial to understand the causes of psychiatric problems. Causes do matter, however. Regardless of whether the discipline is medicine, economics, politics or any field of human endeavour, to solve a problem, it is best to understand its cause.

In 2008 the US Senate Finance Committee, driven by Republican Senator Charles Grassley, began an investigation into the APA because of its financial ties to the pharmaceutical industry.[9] Grassley's probing led to revelations that in 2006 the pharmaceutical industry:

> accounted for about 30 per cent of the association's US$62.5 million in financing. About half of that money went to drug advertisements in psychiatric journals and exhibits at the annual meeting, and the other half to sponsor fellowships, conferences and industry symposiums at the annual meeting.[10]

In 2008 it was revealed that more than half the psychiatrists that developed the DSM-IV received drug company funds.[11]

Thankfully there has been recent recognition of the problem from the top level of the APA by retiring president Dr Steven S. Sharfstein: 'With every new revelation, our credibility with patients has been damaged, and we have to protect that first and foremost...I think we need to review all arrangements between doctors and industry and be very clear about what constitutes a conflict of interest and what does not'.[12] Earlier in 2008 when still APA President, Dr Sharfstein wrote a groundbreaking commentary piece on the relationship between psychiatry and the pharmaceutical industry entitled 'Big Pharma and American Psychiatry: the Good, the Bad, and the Ugly':

> There is widespread concern of the over-medicalization of mental disorders and the overuse of medications. Financial incentives and managed care have contributed to the notion of a 'quick fix' by taking a pill and reducing the emphasis on psychotherapy and psychosocial treatments. There is much evidence that there is less psychotherapy provided by psychiatrists than 10 years ago. This is true despite the strong evidence base that many psychotherapies are effective used alone or in combination with medications...
>
> One of the charges against psychiatry that was discussed in the resultant media coverage (of anti-psychiatry remarks by Tom Cruise) is that many patients are being prescribed the wrong drugs or drugs they don't need. These charges are true, but it is not psychiatry's fault—it is the fault of the broken health care system that the United States appears to be willing to endure...In a time of economic constraint, a 'pill and

an appointment' has dominated treatment. We must work hard to end this situation and get involved in advocacy to reform our health care system from the bottom up.

There are examples of the 'ugly' practices that undermine the credibility of our profession. Drug company representatives will be the first to say that it is the doctors who request the fancy dinners, cruises, tickets to athletic events, and so on. But can we really be surprised that several states have passed laws to force disclosure of these gifts? So-called 'preceptorships' are another example of the 'ugly'; that is, drug companies who pay physicians to allow company reps to sit in on patient sessions allegedly to learn more about care for patients and then advise the doctor on appropriate prescribing. Drug company representatives bearing gifts are frequent visitors to psychiatrists' offices and consulting rooms. We should have the wisdom and distance to call these gifts what they are—kickbacks and bribes.[13]

Although his comments are similar to the abovementioned comments by Fred Gottlieb some twenty-three years prior, Sharfstein's honest appraisal gives hope of a fresh approach, where patient needs are the primary focus of psychiatric practice. In the meantime the Australian psychiatric profession should abandon its slavish devotion to the APA's flawed and commercially compromised DSM-IV.

DSM-V is due to replace DSM-IV in 2012. One of the primary drivers of DSM-IV, Dr Allen Frances, the former chief of Psychiatry at the Duke University Medical Center, has recognised the disastrous consequences of DSM-IV's sloppy diagnostic criteria for ADHD. (See chapter 1.) Dr Frances warned about similar potential for 'false epidemics' like the 'wild over-diagnosis of Attention Deficit Disorder' in the early draft of DSM-V. He cited the example of the proposal to recognise 'Binge Eating Disorder':

> In order to meet the criteria for this proposed diagnosis, a person would need to binge just once a week for 3 months…And my guess is that before very long, maybe 10 per cent of the population would qualify for this diagnosis of binge eating disorder. That means 20 million people and there's no proven treatment for the condition and undoubtedly, lots of people would be getting unnecessary, expensive and often horrible treatments for conditions that really are made up by the people doing the manual without very strong support or need.[14]

Commonsense like that displayed in retrospect by Dr Frances is resulting in a fightback from 'environmental psychiatrists', who believe it is important to understand the family and social circumstances of individuals. They are concerned about the dominance of the 'pill for every ill' approach of biological psychiatry and commercial ties between psychiatry and pharmaceutical companies. Definitely in the 'environmental psychiatry' camp, Dr Peter Breggin believes: 'Psychiatry is more like a two-party political system with the biological and environmental parties constantly vying for power. Biological psychiatry is now the party in power.'[15] Breggin and his fellow proponents of environmental psychiatry need to wrest power from the biological psychiatrists before psychiatry, particularly American psychiatry, is so discredited that it has no future. The great difficulty for environmental psychiatry is that in the short term at least, biological psychiatry is more profitable and convenient than environmental psychiatry. Therein lies the problem.

The Food and Drug Administration

In America, pharmaceutical companies are free to determine who conducts their studies, which studies they publish and which they keep quiet. The pharmaceutical companies use two basic techniques to keep the Food and Drug Administration and the American public in the dark. The first is to completely ignore negative studies. The second is to spin the results of negative findings for the 'primary outcome' – the main question the study was designed to answer – and highlight a positive 'secondary outcome'.[16] Pfizer, the manufacturer of antidepressant Zoloft, conducted five studies for presentation to the FDA:

> The drug seemed to work better than the placebo in two of them. In three other trials, the placebo did just as well at reducing indications of depression. Only the two favorable trials were published, researchers found, and Pfizer discusses only the positive results in Zoloft's literature for doctors.[17]

These tactics are not limited to Pfizer. In 2008 the *Wall Street Journal* highlighted that in the case of seventy-four pharmaceutical company sponsored studies into antidepressants, thirty-seven of thirty-eight favourable studies were published, but the majority of unfavourable (twenty-two of thirty-six) studies were not. Of the fourteen unfavourable studies that were published, 'at least 11 of those studies mischaracterized the results and presented a negative study as positive…In nine (of 11) of the negative studies that were published, the authors simply omitted any mention of the (negative) primary outcome.'[18]

Just as Australian psychiatric practice has followed the lead of the American Psychiatric Association through its slavish adherence to DSM-IV, the Australian drug regulator the Therapeutic Goods Administration has relied heavily on the lead of the FDA. As Peter Breggin puts it: 'To rely on the FDA is in many ways to rely on the drug companies themselves…During the FDA approval process, the drug company designs the research, selects and pays the researchers, and then collects and interprets the data.'[19]

Dr Breggin highlighted specific concerns with the FDA approval of the slow-release formula Ritalin-SR in 1978. The drug trials for the approval of Ritalin-SR lasted fourteen days and compared forty-five children on Ritalin-SR with forty-five on Ritalin. '10 patients on Ritalin-SR and 8 on Ritalin showed adverse effects that weren't there before they started taking the drug.'[20] Despite patients on Ritalin-SR exhibiting worsening behaviour, anxiety, overly quiet and obsessive behaviour, poor appetite, laughing excessively, fidgeting and restless sleep 'none of these [adverse drug reactions] were considered serious'.[21] The study included no placebo group but allowed the drug company

Ciba to compare Ritalin-SR to Ritalin. They were shown to be equally effective and the approval of Ritalin-SR was based on the assumption that Ritalin was effective. When Breggin tried to obtain the original approval documents for Ritalin, the FDA claimed it had lost the original studies that justified Ritalin's initial market approval in 1956.[22]

More recently, concerns have emerged that the FDA has lost the capacity to review the safety of existing drugs and focuses almost exclusively on the rapid approval of new pharmaceutical treatments. The *New York Times* attributes this change to a 1992 agreement, where the pharmaceutical industry:

> promised to give the agency (the FDA) millions – in the 2003 fiscal year, $200 million – but only if the agency spent a specified level of money on new drug approvals...Indeed, the agency now relies almost entirely on the willingness of drug makers to report problems that crop up after a drug has been approved to ensure the safety of the nation's drug supply.[23]

Some critics, including Dr Avorn of the Harvard Medical School, an expert in pharmacoepidemiology and pharmacoeconomics, believe the failings of the FDA were due more to a lack of courage than money.[24] Regardless of the cause American consumers, and because of the reliance of the TGA on the FDA, Australian consumers, have been exposed to significant yet unnecessary risk.

Off Label Prescribing

The inadequate protection offered by the FDA and licensing system is further weakened by 'off label prescribing'. Pharmaceutical companies get approvals from the FDA or TGA for the treatment of conditions within specified guidelines. However, in both the US and Australia, once a drug has been approved physicians are free to prescribe it as they see fit. This frequently occurs and the drug companies profit and are completely immune to liability for any damage caused by this 'off label' use. Many children are prescribed drugs either at doses above the approved dosage, or in combination with contraindicated medications, because of the clinical judgement of reckless prescribers.

Methylphenidate, for example, is not approved for the treatment of children younger than six. In 1995 the 'off label' prescribing of Ritalin was so widespread in the US that the Drug Enforcement Agency (DEA) expressed concern 'that children under the age of six are being treated with methylphenidate contrary to labelling guidelines in the absence of controlled studies suggesting that this is appropriate'. The DEA entered the debate because they considered Ritalin use a possible 'risk factor for substance abuse'.[25]

The drug companies have the best of both worlds: increased sales with no liability for the clinical judgement of individual practitioners. Drug companies obviously deserve protection from liability due to individual rogue prescribers, but the practice of using psychotropic drugs 'off label' is so common that it represents normal practice, and the drug companies must be aware that this is the case.

Stimulant Black Box Warning Debate

In July 2005, reports of adverse cardiovascular and psychiatric events prompted the FDA to convene a Drug Safety Advisory Panel consisting of sixteen of America's top drug safety experts. The experts were provided with details of the adverse event reports and given the brief of designing further research to establish the safety of ADHD drugs. The Drug Safety Advisory Panel was expected to take a baby step by designing more research, but instead it recommended a great leap forward. It said that there was no need to wait for further studies as there was enough available evidence to justify significant product warnings and labelling changes. It unanimously decided to recommend the inclusion of patient guides as well as labelling changes, particularly in regard to the risk of strokes, heart attacks and other adverse cardiovascular events. There was a majority vote to place a 'black box warning' for cardiovascular risks on all ADHD stimulant drugs. A black box warning is the strongest form of warning issued by the FDA about a drug, the step taken just short of removing it from the market.[26]

Several of the Panel members stated that it would be 'inappropriate, unethical behavior' not to disclose that there was significant uncertainty about the safety of the drugs.[27] Part of the evidence was data that both children and adults taking stimulants were roughly four times more likely to have a heart attack and about two and a half times more likely to have a stroke than people who were not taking the drugs. One of the drug safety experts, cardiologist Dr Steven Nissen, said, 'This is out-of-control use of drugs that have profound cardiovascular consequences...We have got a potential public health crisis. I think patients and families need to be made aware of these concerns.'[28] Dr Nissen was talking about prescribers of ADHD stimulants when he said, 'I want to cause people's hands to tremble a little bit before they write that [prescription]. The only way I know how to do that is to put it in a black box.'[29] Panel member and University of Washington biostatistician Thomas Fleming suggested that the risk of heart attack and adverse cardiovascular events might be comparable to those of the arthritis medication Vioxx, now withdrawn from the market.[30]

Not surprisingly, the Drug Safety Advisory Panel's recommendation created considerable debate and was resisted strongly by the drug companies and their allies. Dr Jon A. Shaw, director of Child and Adolescent Psychiatry at the University of Miami School of Medicine, repeated many of the hypothetical aspects of the ADHD mantras as if they were indisputable fact. He stated, 'It's a real medical condition, and it's associated with neurobiological chemical aberrations. Hundreds of studies have shown that psycho-stimulants improve academic performance, social behaviour, relationships.'[31] Dr Karen Ballaban-Gil, a professor of clinical neurology and clinical paediatrics at Albert Einstein College of Medicine and Montefiore Medical Center in New York City responded with the line: 'Nothing is chicken soup except chicken soup.'[32]

Even Dr Thomas Laughren, director of the Division of Psychiatry Products at the FDA's Center for Drug Evaluation and Research, showed no enthusiasm for the FDA's own Drug Safety Advisory Panel's advice. He also used the standard arguments about benefits outweighing the risks of ADHD drugs as the justification for keeping parents in the dark about their dangers. He responded to the call for a black box warning by saying, 'I think it's important not to minimize the benefits of these drugs'[33], and pre-empted the FDA's consideration of the proposed black box warning on stimulants as a whole, stating: 'We don't think anything different needs to be done right now...We think the labelling right now is adequate.'[34] Dr Robert Temple, director of the FDA's Office of Medical Policy agreed: 'We didn't find the sudden death data very persuasive.' This is hardly the language of a regulator whose first priority is consumer safety. Clearly Drs Laughren, Temple and Shaw, on behalf of the FDA – the agency charged with protecting American consumers, including children – had reversed the onus of proof in favour of the drug companies.

Following the Drug Safety Advisory Panel's black box warning recommendation, a paediatric advisory committee of the FDA also issued conflicting recommendations, concluding again that the benefits of medication outweighed any risks. Ultimately, the FDA accepted the arguments of the paediatrics panel over that of the multidisciplinary drug safety experts and strengthened warnings, but did not apply a boxed warning to ADHD stimulants. It is alarming that the FDA followed the advice of paediatricians and ignored that of drug safety experts on an issue of drug safety. The official rationale was that despite the 'complete absence of similar reports in children treated with dummy pills' there was not a 'definitive link between reported psychiatric events and the use of stimulant drugs'.[35] If the FDA is only going to act when there is a 'definitive link' rather than 'high probability' it is unlikely it will ever act to protect children from the possible side effects of ADHD medication.

Antidepressants, a Depressing Precedent

When discussing the decision of the FDA not to follow the Drug Safety Panel's recommendation Dr Laughren was critical of a previous FDA action to protect children. He said, 'We put a black box (for suicidality) on antidepressants for adolescents, but it did have an impact on prescribing and there's been a lot of negative feedback from the clinical community. It's important to recognize that something as dramatic as a black box can have a dramatic effect on prescribing.'[36]

The fact that antidepressants are supposed to 'cheer up' depressed people, but instead increase the risk of suicide poses obvious questions. Dr Laughren's concerns about 'impact on prescribing and negative feedback from the clinical community' invite the question as to whether Laughren and the FDA were more concerned about consumer safety or the profits of the pharmaceutical companies and the happiness of the clinical community.

Friends in High Places

Sometimes the failure of government to regulate effectively is a product of lack of interest and incompetence, but sometimes there is an unhealthy and unethical co-dependence. The most notable case of an improper relationship between government and drug companies was the favouritism extended to Eli Lilly, manufacturer of the non-stimulant ADHD drug Strattera, (see appendix 1) by the former US president George W. Bush. President Bush signed off on restrictions to Eli Lilly's liability for damage to the health of American children, from the inclusion of mercury in Eli Lilly vaccines, when the Homeland Security Bill was passed into law in November 2002. In addition the 'White House had asked a court to keep secret certain documents relating to the vaccine cases involving (Eli) Lilly and a number of other companies.'[37]

These decisions need to be viewed in the light of the long and close relationship between the Bush family and Eli Lilly. George W. Bush's father, former president George H. Bush, was director of Eli Lilly in the 1970s; and when his son was in power a former executive of the company ran the budget office in the White House. In 2002 the company's chair was appointed as an adviser to the president on homeland security.[38] It is difficult to make a legitimate connection between Eli Lilly's potential financial liabilities and US national security. One explanation is that as a favour to family cronies, George W. Bush cynically attached a clause designed to benefit Eli Lilly to the back of legislation supposed to prevent domestic terrorism in the wake of 9/11 that no US politician would oppose.

The Bush family were not the only US politicians to enjoy a close relationship with Eli Lilly. The *Australian Financial Review* said, 'According to the Center for Responsive Politics, Eli Lilly donated more than $3 million to individual election campaigns, 80 per cent of it to Republican candidates, and there are reports the company spent $13 million on lobbying in Washington last year.'[39] In a climate of political patronage governments are far less likely to ensure their regulators rely on thorough, objective, impartial scientific research.

In an interesting twist, on the night George W. Bush was confirmed as the Republican Party's nomination for the 2000 presidential election, his nephew Pierce Bush and Pierce's father

Neil appeared on US national television talk show, *Larry King Live* and talked about Pierce's refusal to take ADHD medication[40]:

> LARRY KING: Neil, tell me about Pierce. Has he always been this way, upfront?
>
> NEIL BUSH (FATHER): Pierce has always been gifted.
>
> LARRY KING: He's not shy.
>
> NEIL BUSH: Clearly, he's not shy. He's an incredibly talented young kid. And let me tell you a personal story, Larry, which is – kind of tell you a little bit about my business. Pierce has been in this school where, despite the fact that he's truly gifted, he's been having – he had a lot of difficulty [in] 6th, 7th and 8th grade. And he was diagnosed by some as ADD and that kind of thing. They tried to put him on Ritalin.
>
> PIERCE BUSH: I wouldn't take it.
>
> NEIL BUSH: Pierce refused to take Ritalin. And so we took him to a place where they did a full assessment, three and a half days, and came to the conclusion that Pierce is a gifted and talented kid. And I mean, it's...
>
> LARRY KING: What were they reading wrong?
>
> NEIL BUSH: Well, the schools today, private schools, public schools, all schools have this boring, you know, lecture in textbook style teaching and that doesn't get the kids like Pierce.

Pierce Bush's experience is the same as many talented and bored students whose uninterested inattention gets diagnosed as ADHD. Most children, however, do not have access to a three-and-a-half-day full assessment and instead retain an ADHD diagnosis and remain on drugs, swelling the profits of pharmaceutical companies like Eli Lilly.

Pierce Bush may be doing well but American children are not. As American psychologist Dr Leonard Sax points out, given that many of the supposed benefits of medication for ADHD children relate to education, 'you would expect American children to be racing ahead in their school work', but as it is, 'France, Germany, and Japan continue to maintain their traditional lead over the United States in tests of math and reading ability'.[41] Similarly, if ADHD drugs worked, measures of social functioning like juvenile crime rates would be lower in countries with high prescribing rates like the US. America should hardly be Australia's role model for enhancing the welfare of children.

5

The Politics of ADHD

Prescribing medication to children diagnosed with ADHD works well for cynical, populist politicians. At a relatively low cost it gives the appearance of addressing children's mental health needs. Even governments that may believe there is something not quite right with giving amphetamines to inattentive children become fearful that if they act decisively, they will alienate parents who have come to depend on subsidised drugs as their chief means of controlling behaviour. This is entirely understandable. There are votes to be lost telling parents that the 'magic bullet' they are giving their 'improved' child is in fact sometimes a crutch propping up their inadequate parenting or simply a mask hiding a host of other more complex problems.

Most governments leave the issue of ADHD in the too hard basket. Typical of this timid approach was former Western Australian health minister Kevin Prince's response in 1997 to a parliamentary question regarding the state government's attitude to ADHD. Despite Western Australia then having four times the national rate of PBS-subsidised dexamphetamine prescriptions, Minister Prince said: '[ADHD] is a matter that should be addressed on a nationwide basis and it should not be taken up by one State to the exclusion of all others, because it clearly affects the totality of Australian people'.[1] Minister Prince's almost comical desire to pass the buck to another level of government reflects in *Yes, Minister* terms how 'courageous' it is to express a view on this issue. When responsible governments rise to this challenge they naturally have one eye on the public good and the other on the ballot box. Good governments express concern about misdiagnosis and over-prescription. None are ever brave enough to say ADHD is a fraud.

Since 2003 successive Western Australian governments have been as interventionist as any in reducing ADHD prescribing rates to children. In 2003 controls on prescribing clinicians were tightened. (See chapter 6.) In 2004 a Western Australian parliamentary inquiry into ADHD changed the course of public debate and in November 2009, the first of two multidisciplinary clinics to treat children with problems of attention was opened in Joondalup, a northern suburb of Perth. These clinics were first promised by the then premier Alan Carpenter in September 2007, who when announcing funding for them told state parliament that:

> Although medication may still be required for severe cases of ADHD, this new approach will ensure that stimulant medication is not the first line of treatment... The aim is to reduce the prescription rates for young people suffering ADHD. If our recent history is any

guide, reducing ADHD prescription rates will reduce amphetamine abuse rates, and we all know that the abuse and misuse of amphetamines is a major issue in our society broadly.[2]

I scripted Carpenter's statement, fully aware that if a significant political leader made too strong a statement there may have been a backlash from parents who had come to rely on stimulants.

Even my own advocacy on ADHD has, until recently, been tempered by the reality that parents with children on ADHD medication vote, and if I tell the whole brutal truth they may not vote for me. In truth, I consider parents at best desperate, vulnerable and gullible, and at worst reckless, in regard to the long-term wellbeing of their child. When lobbying both state and federal governments, however, I have tried to position the government to be concerned about prescription rates, and to support strategies designed to ensure medications are not the first and only line of treatment. This pragmatic approach shifts government policy to a less pro-drug position; however, it leaves the door open for prescribing children amphetamines and implicitly recognises the validity of ADHD, even if as a diagnosis of last resort.

I believe in the next five to ten years medicating children for ADHD will be seen as a tragic abuse of their rights, and society will collectively wonder how it all happened. Democratically elected governments rarely get ahead of public opinion, however, and for the moment getting them to support strategies aimed at making ADHD medications a last order treatment is a good result. No government will ban the use of amphetamines by children until it is no longer brave to do so.

The NHMRC

The National Health and Medical Research Council (NHMRC) is an independent statutory agency funded by the Commonwealth government to develop recommendations for best health policy and practice. The NHMRC typically outsources development of treatment guidelines and other research to individuals and organisations with the relevant expertise. In 1997 the NHMRC outsourced the production of comprehensive and influential guidelines designed to advise clinicians on the diagnosis and treatment of ADHD. The main message from the 1997 NHMRC guidelines to clinicians was clear: 'medication can work similarly across the range of cognitive ability and age'.[3] If a patient was young or old, bright or dull, if they had difficulty organising their life and were inclined to act on impulse or were inattentive, stimulants were the answer.

Furthermore, the 1997 guidelines encouraged clinicians to diagnose outside DSM-IV criteria and prescribe outside approved guidelines if the diagnosis complied 'with reasonable theory'.[4] What constituted 'reasonable theory' was not specified; it was left to the clinician to determine. Prescribing for any behaviour that could possibly be caused by a 'biochemical imbalance' or even just modified by 'medication', clearly, in the mind of many clinicians, constituted 'reasonable theory'. This freedom was reinforced by the statement that 'clinical experience may precede research', which further encouraged clinicians, particularly those with an inflated sense of their own ability, to prescribe ahead of research.[5]

The badge of the NHMRC gave this report legitimacy and contributed to the national prescribing explosion of the 1990s that continues today. The NHMRC sensibly decided that the 1997 guidelines were not sufficiently evidence-based, and they were rescinded on 31 December 2005.

The Replacement National Guidelines

The development of replacement guidelines was outsourced by the NHMRC, at a cost of $135,000, to the Royal Australasian College of Physicians (RACP).[6] Far from being an independent guardian of professional standards, the RACP benefits from considerable sponsorship from drug manufacturers. For example, the RACP 2009 Annual Physicians Week Conference was sponsored by ADHD drug manufacturer Janseen–Cilag and had paid exhibitions by Eli Lilly and Novartis. On the RACP website, potential sponsors and exhibitors were encouraged to fund the RACP Conference with comments like 'Sponsorship and Exhibition opportunities allow you to align the needs of your company to specific Congress events, whilst exposing your staff directly to your captive target markets [i.e. prescribers].'[7]

Rather than being addressed, the deficiencies of the rescinded 1997 guidelines were reinforced. The RACP guidelines committee was initially chaired by Dr Daryl Efron until his drug company ties were exposed by the *Daily Telegraph* in April 2007 – he had been on the advisory boards of Novartis (Ritalin) and Eli Lilly (Strattera). When confronted by the newspaper, Dr Efron argued his drug company ties were irrelevant, stating, 'the important thing is we declare our potential conflicts of interest'.[8] He revealed the extent of his enthusiasm for medicating children diagnosed ADHD by declaring he supported the use of

Ritalin by children under the age of six despite the manufacturer recommending against it.[9]

Abbott Leaves It to the 'Experts'

Media exposure of Dr Efron's pharmaceutical company ties prompted then health minister Tony Abbott's intervention and Efron's resignation as chair, but not from the committee. Abbott said he 'instinctively questioned' the long-term use of drugs for non–life-threatening conditions.[10] This followed comments the previous week by then prime minister John Howard who said, 'I am very worried about reports of the over-prescription of Ritalin.'[11] These were admirable sentiments; however, the fatal flaw in the Howard government's approach was revealed in minister Abbott's qualifying statement: 'I want to see new clinical guidelines but I stress it is up to the *experts* to carefully weigh all the issues.'[12] (Emphasis added.) The problem is, apart from a few determined and isolated sceptics, the 'experts' in ADHD are almost exclusively fervent believers in the validity of the diagnosis and the safety and effectiveness of the drugs. Sceptics are generally not motivated to specialise or become 'expert' in conditions they don't believe in. It is not easy to make an income from specialising in 'not' diagnosing a condition. On the other hand there are substantial incentives, both commercial and professional, for 'true believers' in ADHD to become experts. No sceptics made it onto the RACP guidelines panel, only 'true believers'. Abbott had delegated the solution to the problem of reckless prescribing to those who had created it in the first place.

Roxon's Hypocrisy

When Dr Efron's ties were exposed, the then opposition health spokesperson and current Minister for Health, Nicola Roxon, railed about protecting kids from unnecessary prescribing.[13] Roxon demanded transparency and called for the names and drug company connections of the guidelines review committee members to be made public, saying, 'These guidelines are incredibly important and it is important there is public confidence in them. Given the controversy surrounding ADHD, releasing the names is the sensible option to help restore public confidence in the process.'[14] Abbott rejected Roxon's call for full disclosure.

But when in November 2007 Roxon became Minister of Health, she failed to disclose the names of the committee or their drug company connections. If it were not for Freedom of Information processes, the public wouldn't have known about committee members' commercial ties to drug companies. In November 2008 the Adelaide *Advertiser* revealed that:

> Seven of the original 10 [guidelines committee] group members, including doctors, have declared receiving grants and air fares, hotels and overseas trips from companies making drugs to treat the disorder. One non-medical member, former teacher Geraldine Moore, had the bill for her Sydney book launch picked up by Eli Lilly, manufacturer of one of the two major ADHD drugs, Stattera…The newsaper has obtained the conflict of interest declarations made by nine of

the 10 original working group members. The 10th has demanded details remain secret. Two of the nine since have quit. Among replacements is educational consultant Michelle Pearce, who helped write a booklet 'Teenagers with ADHD' for drug company, Novartis.[15]

When the *Advertiser* ran its article, it was reported that 'the publicly-funded committee had threatened to quit if their names were revealed'.[16] Instead of continuing to allow the connections to be hidden, Minister Roxon should have welcomed their resignations and appointed replacements who didn't take drug company money. Adelaide psychiatrist and campaigner against ADHD prescribing, Dr Jon Jureidini, said many doctors had said no to drug company money and would have been well qualified to join the committee adding, 'It is incredibly easy not to accept the money, you just decide not to do it.'[17]

Following up on the *Advertiser* article, independent South Australian Senator Nick Xenophon asked for details of potential conflicts of interest. The response: 'Minister [Roxon] has been advised that the conflicts of interest declared by working party members are consistent with the normal range associated with clinician review committees of this nature.'[18] If seven out of ten members having pharmaceutical company connections is within 'the normal range associated with clinician review committees of this nature' then there are obvious questions about the independence of these review committee processes. Certainly the Commonwealth government should not be relying on them as a source of 'independent expert' advice.

In addition to calling for full committee disclosure when

in opposition, Roxon also called for an independent inquiry into ADHD 'along the lines of one into ADHD in Western Australia'.[19] Shadow minister Roxon (unlike Minister Roxon) had wanted the inquiry to address the community's 'clear' concern that Australia has one of the world's highest rates of ADHD prescribing, stating, 'we don't want children being medicated if they don't need to be and we want to make sure children who need support and assistance can get it, so we must get the balance right'.[20] The Australian Medical Association's response to Roxon's call was to protect the interests of their membership by defending prescribing practices, rejecting a 'full-blown inquiry' and insisting the RACP committee complete its work.[21]

The Western Australian inquiry Roxon referred to was conducted in 2004 by six parliamentarians: four from the Labor Party (including me as a co-opted, non-voting member), one from the Liberal Party and one from the National Party, none of whom had any commercial interest in ADHD. (See chapter 6.) While I had a predetermined position on ADHD and one other member Paul Andrews MLA, like me a former teacher, had privately expressed concern about ADHD prescribing, none of the other four members, including the chair Carol Martin MLA or the deputy chair Mike Board MLA, had any past experience of the issue. The parliamentary inquiry reached unanimous conclusions. In contrast, the RACP guidelines review was conducted by a group of drug company allies, with a clear commercial and professional investment in the continued medicating of children for ADHD. Despite her earlier praise for the Western Australian parliamentary inquiry, since becoming Minister for Health Nicola Roxon has ignored the lessons that can be learned from WA. She has taken the powerful

AMA's advice and relied on the conflicted RACP guidelines review group.

One of the few guideline committee members not to have drug company connections was Dr Efron's replacement as chairman, Western Australian paediatrician Dr David Forbes. Eighteen months after taking the job Dr Forbes defended the drug company connections of the other committee members stating, 'There is absolutely no concern raised that any person on the working group has in any way acted inappropriately and I have every confidence in their professionalism.'[22] It has never been claimed that guidelines panel members were acting inappropriately by accepting hidden kickbacks or deliberately hiding drug company connections. Yet despite Dr Forbes's assurance of professionalism, the RACP guidelines committee cannot be regarded as independent or free of pro-pharmaceutical company bias. Predictably the committee came up with draft recommendations that, if implemented, will swell both the numbers of children on ADHD drugs and pharmaceutical company profits.

Perhaps the most revealing element of the draft guidelines was that two thirds of the recommendations were made without any supporting scientific evidence. They were based entirely on reference group consensus and justified as 'best practice based on clinical experience and expert opinion'. Like the 2002 International Consensus Statement (see chapter 1), these recommendations were made by a group of fervent believers in the validity of ADHD, most of whom had commercial ties to the pharmaceutical industry.

Roxon's Missed Opportunity

Throughout 2009, Roxon came under pressure from both sides of the ADHD debate. Along with others concerned about the potential of the new guidelines to further accelerate the growth in child prescribing rates, I lobbied Roxon to abandon the compromised draft guidelines and seek advice from psychiatrists without ties to the pharmaceutical industry. ADHD proponents, including members of the RACP guidelines committee, wanted the guidelines to be released.

In November 2009 the NHMRC effectively offered Roxon an ideal circuit breaker. They announced that because of an investigation involving undisclosed drug company payments to US researcher Dr Joseph Biederman, the guidelines had not been approved and that 'If the US investigation remains unresolved by mid-2010, NHMRC will move to redevelop the draft guidelines'.[23] To my surprise and dismay Roxon rejected this opportunity to defuse the issue and pressured the NHMRC to release the guidelines. The public and the medical profession were left with the mixed message that according to the NHMRC the guidelines were draft and subject to withdrawal, but that Roxon was pleased they finally offered 'more up-to-date information on ways to identify and care for those in our community who may be suffering from ADHD'.[24] This was not the only inconsistency in the Commonwealth government's response.

Roxon, the RACP and the NHMRC claimed in a joint press release that there were over 350,000[25] Australian children and adolescents with ADHD (over seven times the number medicated in 2007).[26] Yet the RACP guidelines chair Dr Forbes stated 'What's important is that it is likely fewer children will be prescribed medication.'[27]

The incompetence of the RACP guidelines panel was fully revealed when a spokesperson asserted that 'the College was not aware of the US investigation (into Biederman) when drafting the guidelines'.[28] As was revealed in the *Australian* the day after the RACP made this claim, I 'wrote to the panel in July last year, [sixteen months earlier] warning that its work had been tainted by Dr Biederman's research' and 'raised similar concerns with Ms Roxon's advisers in August last year'.[29] My submission to the RACP guidelines committee stated:

> On June 8 2008 the *New York Times* exposed how Dr Biederman was paid US$1.6 million in consulting fees from drug makers between 2000 and 2007 but did not disclose this income to his employer Harvard University.[30] Biederman received research funds from 15 pharmaceutical companies and serves as a paid speaker or adviser to at least seven drug companies.[31]

My submission was obviously ignored. Regardless of their inattention to my submissions, if the RACP committee or Roxon's office had been monitoring developments in the ADHD debate, they would have known about the Biederman scandal. With a little further research they would have also found that Dr Biederman was not the only Harvard University researcher cited in the draft guidelines under investigation for undisclosed drug company payments. Two other Harvard researchers under investigation, Drs Timothy Wilens and Thomas Spencer, were cited thirty-two and forty-six times respectively.[32] The practice of hiding drug company payments may not be restricted to Harvard. At least two other researchers cited in the guidelines,

Drs Karen Wagner and Augustus John Rush of the University of Texas, were also under investigation for similar misconduct.[33]

Another researcher cited on twenty-five occasions was Dr Laurence Greenhill, who co-authored a number of the referenced studies. Dr Greenhill has worked as a paid consultant to Alza Corp., Bristol-Myers Squibb, Richwood and GlaxoSmithKline, Eli Lilly, McNeil Pharmaceutical, Novartis Pharmaceuticals and Solvay.[34] He has been a paid speaker for ADHD drug manufacturers Eli Lilly, Janssen Pharmaceuticals and Novartis Pharmaceuticals.[35] When addressing an audience of 300 international psychiatrists at a conference in Melbourne in September 2006, Dr Greenhill misrepresented the FDA deliberations on the black box warning debate on stimulants.[36] (See chapter 4.) He portrayed the call for a black box warning for stimulants as coming from isolated clinicians rather than from the specially appointed FDA Drug Safety Advisory Panel. Dr Greenhill only revealed his extensive drug company connections when I asked him about them at the end of his presentation.

In addition to relying on compromised researchers, the draft guidelines document highlighted that 'the majority of the identified studies on ADHD medications have been sponsored, at least in part, by the manufacturers of the medications'.[37] Nonetheless, these typically extreme short-term studies were used to support ADHD drugs as a 'first line treatment'. Predictably, they demonstrated that nothing alters behaviour faster than behaviour-altering drugs. Furthermore, compelling evidence that there are no sustained benefits, only significant risks, from long-term exposure to these toxins was either downplayed or ignored. Despite my personally offering a copy of the Oregon Health and Science University, *Drug Class Review on Pharmacologic*

Treatments for ADHD to committee chairperson Dr David Forbes and including a summary of it in my submission, this valuable analysis into the safety and efficacy of ADHD drugs was ignored.[38] The result of this biased, compromised process is that, despite Dr Forbes's claim to the contrary, the upward spiral in Australian ADHD prescribing rates will continue unabated, if these guidelines are followed.

What Harm Will Be Done?

The key recommendations of the draft guidelines encourage the use of stimulants, either methylphenidate or dexamphetamine, with the substitution of one for the other in the case of adverse side effects or ineffectiveness. If children do 'not respond to or are intolerant of stimulant medication', the non-stimulant drug Strattera is recommended. (See appendix 1.)[39] If both stimulants and Strattera fail to result in a 'clinical response' Clonidine can be 'trialled'.[40] This cascading use of medications, without stopping to give children a chance to be chemical-free, causes them damage. An example of this approach is the recommendation that if, as is common, ADHD stimulants cause tics or preexisting tics become worse, the following treatment options can be followed:

1. continue the ADHD medication alone;
2. add an anti-tic medication; or
3. trial another ADHD medication.[41]

The guidelines also encourage polypharmacy, by prescribing a range of psychotropic drugs to children, particularly for depression and bipolar disorder along with ADHD medications. This is despite the TGA insisting manufacturers of all selective serotonin reuptake inhibitors (SSRI) antidepressants include advice that their use by under-twenty-four-year-olds increases the risk of suicidality.[42] Similarly, the recommendation that methylphenidate be used as a second line treatment for children under six years of age, despite manufacturers' guidelines stating otherwise, exposes very young children to significant risks and prescribers to potential negligence claims.[43]

The draft guidelines included numerous statements like:

> the dominant current paradigm suggests that disordered fronto-striato-cerebellar brain circuitry underpins the executive function deficits at the core of this condition. Twin studies have established a strong genetic component. This appears to involve polymorphisms in a number of genes, including those coding for dopamine transporters.[44]

These 'suggestions' and 'appearances' are assumed to be sufficient evidence of a biochemical brain imbalance. As for the genetic basis of ADHD being supported by twin studies, it is obvious that personality traits like distractibility and hyperactivity are in part determined by genetics; however, difference is not disease.

Given the bias of the participants it is not surprising that they concluded 'the use of stimulant medication to treat people with ADHD does not increase the risk of developing substance use disorder'.[45] What is ignored, however, is the blindingly obvious: that methylphenidate and dexamphetamine are controlled substances (Schedule 8 drugs) precisely because they are drugs of addiction with a high potential for abuse. Again in my submission to the RACP and in a letter to Roxon, I provided details of the Western Australian experience of a huge fall in ADHD prescribing rates for children, which coincided with the massive fall in teenage amphetamine abuse rates. Again this evidence was ignored.

The role and rights of parents and family in the draft guidelines are of particular concern. The recommendation that stimulants can be used even on preschoolers if ADHD symptoms are having a severe impact on 'family/carers' is a violation of the rights of the child.[46] Children must never be medicated for the benefit of third parties. Claims of improved family functioning or similar third party benefits must be ignored. The only consideration should be the long-term wellbeing of the individual child. Not the parent, not the teacher, not the classroom, but the child.

An earlier draft of the guidelines included the recommendation that 'Federal, State and Territory funding allocations to schools need to be revised to enable schools to access funding for students diagnosed with ADHD'.[47] This would, if implemented, have provided a commission-based ADHD spotters' fee to schools. This has been the experience in the US where there has been an explosion in ADHD drugging rates partly driven by schools seeking desperately needed general purpose funds.[48] In 1991 the US Department of Education issued a memorandum setting guidelines for schools with children diagnosed ADHD to be made eligible for a special subsidy of approximately US$420 per child per year, under the health impaired category. Children 'may get little more than the services of a nurse or clerk handing out a dose of Ritalin while the money goes into a general purpose fund'.[49]

Fortunately, after a letter from a group of fourteen researchers in education, disabilities and ADHD (led by Dr Linda Graham) to the Rudd government gained media coverage, this recommendation was dropped. The letter criticised 'moves to instruct teachers to look out for ADHD and to allocate special funding to schools for students with the disorder'.[50]

Other equally disturbing recommendations, however, remained in the final draft. The recommendation that 'as ADHD and ADHD symptoms are common in individuals entering the justice system, screening for ADHD may be indicated in this population'[51] carries the risk of prisons being awash with diverted ADHD amphetamines. Like the majority of the 208 recommendations, this was based entirely on the consensus of the RACP panel with no supporting evidence. The admission in the guidelines that 'more research is needed to determine whether treatment of ADHD can reduce the risk of crime and recidivism' simply highlights that bias is the basis of the prison screening proposal.[52]

Even more worrying is the recommendation that 'given the high rate of suicide in Australia's Indigenous population and the association of impulsivity with suicidal ideation among Indigenous youth…there is an urgent need for culturally appropriate assessment of ADHD.'[53]

Fortunately, although there are some notable exceptions, ADHD prescribing rates in non-metropolitan Aboriginal communities are generally below the Australian average. This must not change. The last thing that Aboriginal communities need is a source of cheap amphetamines.

Perhaps the most disturbing potential outcome of the guidelines affects people with intellectual disabilities. They are among the most vulnerable members of society. The recommendation that 'in people with intellectual disability and ADHD, use of stimulant medication should be considered' reflects an absurd expectation of 'normal' for children with intellectual disability.[54] The 'clear evidence of clinically significant impairment in social, academic or occupational functioning' required for a DSM–IV diagnosis is a result of their intellectual impairment not ADHD.[55] Children and adults with intellectual disabilities need a safe, loving, interesting environment, not more labels and amphetamines.

Roxon has allowed the response to concerns about mis-diagnosis and over-prescription to remain delegated to the ADHD industry. The Howard and Rudd governments made the same mistake in seeking to address concerns about reckless prescription. They kept going back to the ADHD industry for advice and the industry inevitably promotes further pre-scribing. Western Australian governments, initially Labor and now Liberal, only made progress on tackling the state's out of control child prescribing rates when they stopped listening to ADHD proponents. It is a pity Canberra is not prepared to learn from Perth's experience.

Economic Bias

The Commonwealth government has created an economic bias towards the diagnosis of ADHD and the related pharmaco-logical interventions. It currently subsidises dexamphetamine (since 1992), Ritalin (2005), Ritalin LA, Concerta and Strattera (2007). Subsidising drugs through the Pharmaceutical Benefits

Scheme encourages their use as the first and often only line of treatment. In addition, un-timed Medicare co-payments mean that paediatricians receive the same financial reward for a rushed or comprehensive consultation. Along with inadequate subsidies for allied health treatment (for example speech and occupational therapy), this encourages the speedy diagnosis of ADHD rather than a full assessment of a child's real needs.

In some Australian states extra in-class support is provided to students with a range of diagnosed disabilities. While a diagnosis of ADHD does not qualify for extra in-class support, parents of a child diagnosed with ADHD may be entitled to a fortnightly Commonwealth carer allowance of $87.30 (in 2008).[56] By contrast in Finland, '"diagnoses" do not fulfil the gate-keeping function…every student who needs it is entitled to additional assistance. There, results indicating poor academic achievement act as a barometer indicating the need for additional support.[57] Surely it makes sense for schools to concentrate their resources on students whose failure to thrive is evidenced by poor results compared to their peers, rather than via increasingly subjective notions of 'disability'?

What Should the Australian Government Do?

In an ideal world where children's interests were paramount and politics irrelevant the Commonwealth government could immediately:

1. Follow the World Health Organization (WHO) and shun the American Psychiatric Association by only providing

financial support (including Medicare co-payments and PBS drug subsidisation) for the treatment of mental health disorders diagnosed using the WHO's more rigorous ICD-10 criteria. Australia is a member of the WHO but has no capacity to influence the American Psychiatric Association's DSM–IV. Why should our psychiatric profession continue to cede sovereignty to the home of pharmaceutical company driven psychiatry?

2. End the PBS subsidisation of amphetamines use for under-eighteens and redirect the savings to treatments that actually help children like speech therapy, occupational therapy and extra in-class support.

3. Restrict PBS subsidisation of psychotropic drugs for children to those initially prescribed and thereafter supervised by child psychiatrists. Only child psychiatrists receive the comprehensive training in mental health and pharmacology required to understand the complexities of childhood behaviours and the limitations of medications. Paediatricians and GPs don't have the same depth of training. Allowing these non-experts to prescribe is a big part of the reason for the explosion in child prescribing rates for bipolar disorder, anxiety, depression and ADHD in children.[58] While there are exceptions, in my experience child psychiatrists are generally less free with their prescription pad than non-experts who dabble in psychiatry. Making the practice of child psychiatry the exclusive right of child psychiatrists would give the profession the chance to get its house in order by imposing appropriate consistent standards.

4. Fund the nationwide replication of Western Australia's Stimulants Monitoring system for all Schedule 8 drugs on

the condition that no member of the monitoring panel is a frequent prescriber or has ties to the pharmaceutical industry. External scrutiny was the main reason Western Australian prescribing rates for children fell. (See chapter 6.) It worked once and it can work again.

5. Beef up Consumer Medicine Information (CMI) requirements so that every warning currently included in information to prescribers is also on the CMI. Prescribing doctors should also be obliged by law to hand patients or parents a CMI, and it should be compulsory to insert CMI sheets in medication packaging.

6. Put black box warnings on the outside packaging of drugs as with cigarette packaging so consumers are aware of very significant risks. Currently black box warnings are often only highlighted on prescriber's information and are never seen by consumers.

7. Require full public disclosure of pharmaceutical industry funding sources for clinicians, researchers, patient groups, advisory board members etc. Parents and patients are entitled to know what factors other than patient welfare might be motivating the doctors and patient support groups that are advising them. Likewise, government and the public are entitled to know about the commercial ties of researchers and advisers.

8. Provide full public disclosure of documents supporting successful applications to approve or subsidise medications. With the exception of unique intellectual property, there should be full public disclosure of the information used to determine that drugs are safe and effective or that are to be subsidised via our taxes.

9. Outlaw pharmaceutical company donations to political parties and candidates and compensate if necessary through increased public funding of political parties. Governments are responsible for multi-million-dollar decisions about which drugs get approved and subsidised and must make these decisions without fear or favour. While a similar case could be made for a range of industries, the pharmaceutical industry is unique in that it produces mind- and body-altering chemicals that are ingested by children. Many of these chemical interventions are lifesaving; most are warranted but as with ADHD some are highly questionable. Government must be free from improper influence of the pharmaceutical industry.

10. Make adverse drug event reporting for a specified range of serious reactions (suicidal ideation, strokes, psychosis) mandatory and regularly publish full details on the web. Voluntary reporting means that only a tiny fraction of adverse events ever get reported, partly because it is in the interest of reckless prescribers not to report serious adverse events. The public has a right to know and policy makers need to know so they can make informed decisions about the risk benefit profile of medications.

11. Prevent doctor shopping and pharmacy shopping for frequently abused drugs by enabling better sharing of patient prescribing information and replicating Western Australian and New South Wales requirements that repeat scripts of Schedule 8 drugs be held by a single pharmacist.

Some of the abovementioned strategies, particularly in relation to disclosure and informed consent, are virtually cost-free and could be implemented without political risk. Others require direct Commonwealth government intervention in the pattern of medical practice and, while warranted, are fraught with political risks. Vested interests, notably non-expert prescribers, the pharmaceutical industry, patient support groups and some parents would resist measures that restrict easy access to psychotropic drugs for children.

To minimise these political risks the government could do what it has always done and outsource the development of policy. The difference being, this time it must outsource to psychiatrists who favour non-drug interventions as the first line response to childhood behavioural problems. This is what Tony Abbott should have done in 2007 when Dr Daryl Efron's drug company ties were exposed. It is what Nicola Roxon should have allowed to happen in 2009 when the NHMRC offered her the opportunity. It is what I asked Kevin Rudd to do when I wrote to him in April 2010, but he ignored my request. Hopefully subsequent governments will succeed where the Rudd and Howard governments have failed. It is still not too late; it is always better late than never.

6

The Rise and Fall of ADHD in Western Australia

Perth is the most isolated capital city in the world with two thousand kilometres of desert separating the city from its nearest neighbour Adelaide. This isolation has shaped Perth's character and it tends to act independently of eastern Australia. Until 2005 Perth had one medical school and still has a cliquey medical community that, at least publicly, is reluctant to criticise its colleagues. This lack of a critical culture allowed a handful of clinicians to dominate clinical practice and led to an explosion in child prescription rates for ADHD. Perth's ADHD story contains the key disturbing elements of the global debate. But the story also offers hope that with commonsense and leadership, spiralling prescribing rates can be turned around.

WA's ADHD History: Key Statistics

In 1989 in WA, 880 people were prescribed stimulant medication. By 2000 there were 20,648 Western Australians on prescription stimulants. The Western Australian Health Department estimated 85 to 90 per cent (17,551 to 18,583) were children.[1] This represented 4.2 per cent to 4.5 per cent of all Western Australian children aged between 4–17 years.[2] Total prescription numbers continued to grow until late 2003 when there was a massive downturn, and by 2005, 8057 children were on stimulants.[3] Child prescribing rates continued to fall and by 2008 only 5666 children were on stimulants.[4] Over a similar time period (2002–08) there was a massive 58 per cent decline in teenage amphetamine abuse rates, supporting the commonsense assertion that prescribing amphetamines facilitates their abuse.[5]

1989–2003: Perth's ADHD Epidemic

From 1989 to 2003 Western Australia saw a massive increase in ADHD prescribing rates – by 2003 the per capita prescribing rates were approximately three times the Australian average.[6] There is limited data available, but it appears the disproportionate rates were due both to higher per capita patient rates and higher than average doses. WA's per capita prescribing rates were comparable with the highest in the world until the state government stopped listening to the ADHD industry and intervened to protect children.[7] Despite fervent criticism from the pro-medication camp, controls on prescribing amphetamines were tightened in 2003, and in 2004 a parliamentary inquiry triggered an intense local debate about the validity of the diagnosis and the safety of the drugs. Since 2003, prescriptions for children have plummeted while they have skyrocketed in all other states. Although WA still has the highest (and rising) adult prescribing rates in Australia, Perth gave up its claim to be the ADHD child prescribing capital of Australia. Sydney, Brisbane and Hobart now vie for that dubious honour.

In 2004 when giving evidence to the Western Australian Parliament Education and Health Standing Committee Inquiry into ADHD, Dr Trevor Parry, a senior Perth paediatrician and former clinical associate professor at the University of Western Australia School of Paediatrics and Child Health, said:

> There was a time in WA history – now fortunately concluded – in which one or two prescribers were following a pattern of prescribing...that was not the gold standard model which most of us believed in... That caused a skewing of over-prescribing within certain locations in the metropolitan area...There was a professional glitch in the system, I guess, that we believe has now fortunately been addressed.[8]

Although Dr Parry did not name him, it is possible that one of the prescribers referred to was paediatrician Dr Harry Nash. Dr Nash had moved from Adelaide in 1999 following complaints about the quality of his diagnostic and prescribing practices.[9] Nash left Perth and returned to the city of Adelaide in 2001. In 2005 Nash's prescribing habits were spectacularly exposed when he was interviewed on the popular television show *Sixty Minutes* and revealed that he had prescribed twelve pills a day to an eleven-year-old Adelaide boy. This was despite a South Australian law preventing the prescription of more than six dexamphetamine pills to children without a second medical opinion.

MIKE MUNRO: You don't think that dexamphetamine and Ritalin are over-prescribed?

DR HARRY NASH: In actual fact, I think they're under-prescribed.

MIKE MUNRO: Deb Aldridge's eleven-year-old son Challend takes at least twelve pills every day.

DEB ALDRIDGE: Okay, in the morning time, we've got five dexamphetamines. And that is for the ADHD. We've got a Catapres and that's the calming agent. And then we've got the Risperidone, which is for the Tourette's, the tics. Then at one o'clock, he has got three dexs. At 3.15, he's got half a dex, a Catapres and a Risperidone.

MIKE MUNRO: After he's home from school?

DEB ALDRIDGE: Home from school. Then at bedtime, about eight, eight-thirty, he's got two Endep for sleeping disorder.

MIKE MUNRO: A cocktail of drugs to treat a range of conditions – ADHD, anxiety, obsessive compulsive disorder and Tourette's syndrome. Challend faces the prospect of being medicated like this for many years to come...

Back in the Aldridge household, Challend's breakfast is a crumpet followed by five dexamphetamines, one

Catapres and a half a Risperidone, all prescribed by Dr Harry Nash. But such multiple doses are controversial and possibly illegal. To protect children from over-prescription, South Australia introduced a law prohibiting doctors from prescribing over six dexamphetamine a day unless there was a second medical opinion. The law says you've got to get a second opinion.

Dr Harry Nash: Right.

Mike Munro: Did you?

Dr Harry Nash: Mike, I can't remember.

Mike Munro: It's important that you know whether you got a second opinion for an eleven-year-old boy on eight psychiatric drugs a day.

Dr Harry Nash: Mike, I have to check the records. This just came in last year, Mike. So I don't know exactly...Is this being recorded?

Mike Munro: We are recording this, yes.

Dr Harry Nash: Oh, God. You've got me...

Mike Munro: Thousands of files, thousands of patients over the years?

Dr Harry Nash: Yes, that's right, Mike...

Mike Munro: In Harry Nash's case, more than a dozen complaints claiming over-prescription have now seen him close his Adelaide practice. And now that Dr Nash has closed up shop, what are you going to do?

Deb Aldridge: I don't know. To be honest with you, the moment we had to leave, I cried all the way home. I've never met another doctor like him that really, really understands what we were going through. So now all I've got to do is just go to my GP and just hope that she will follow up and prescribe the medications. And if not, I'm just going to have to go on another long, hard search to find another person like Harry Nash.[10]

Nash may have contributed to the problem of over-prescription in Perth, though he was by no means a major cause of the problem. Prescribing rates had been escalating for years before Dr Nash moved to Perth and continued to climb after he returned to Adelaide. Parry's reference to two rogue prescribers causing 'a skewing of over-prescribing within certain locations in the metropolitan area' only portrayed a small part of the picture. As he later acknowledged, the prescribing practices of paediatricians trained by Dr Parry contributed significantly to WA's disproportionately high prescribing rates. Parry, along with other Perth ADHD proponents, argued rates were higher because Western Australian prescribers were better at recognising and diagnosing ADHD than those of other states. Ironically, Parry's proud acceptance of his leading role in spiralling rates occurred when child prescribing rates were in sharp decline. The following transcript is from Channel Nine's *Sunday* program:

REPORTER: One very influential WA paediatrician Trevor Parry says there's no problem with the state's prescription rates.

DR TREVOR PARRY: I have always been happy with that, despite what the critics have said about Western Australia being the drug capital of Australia.

REPORTER: Parry has had a lot to do with the rates of prescription...since he trained many of those practising in the field...You may be practising less but those people you trained are out there following your lead.

DR TREVOR PARRY: I can only hope so!

REPORTER: Western Australia also sits apart from the rest of Australia because doctors here prescribed the medication for ADHD in higher doses...

DR TREVOR PARRY: People are comfortable that up to ten or twelve tablets a day for a certain weight of children...we don't faint and beat our breasts about that if four a day...for high school children is higher than the other states are using then I would hope that for some children other states might become a bit more confident.[11]

Dr Parry often appeared to have a moderate position on ADHD; however, in 2004 he told the Western Australian parliamentary inquiry that children with ADHD 'lookalikes', such as victims of 'child abuse' and 'poor attachment' may also benefit from 'medication'.[12] Unlike Dr Nash, Dr Parry is a respected mainstream practitioner and recent recipient of the Children and Young People Lifetime Achievement Award (part of the WA Citizen of the Year Awards). His very controversial belief is that rather than Western Australia being guilty of misdiagnosing and over-prescribing, the other states were yet to catch up with WA 'best practice'. Parry was refering to Victoria's prescribing rates, when in 2002, he said '[Victorian rates] have been the lowest...because they have not strongly believed in the existence of ADHD nor have they trained their paediatricians accordingly until quite recently'.[13]

Victorian psychiatrist Dr George Halasz put forward an alternative analysis of Western Australia's prescribing rates. Halasz agreed with Parry that differences in training and medical culture accounted for the difference between Western Australian and Victorian prescription rates, yet he was highly critical of Western Australian practice. Halasz believes the increase in ADHD prescription was a consequence of the 'dumbing down' of child mental health assessment, diagnosis and treatment, stating 'the art and science of the assessment of child behaviour had become merely the chronicling of a set of symptoms'.[14] In his opinion this erosion was in part due to the way new doctors were trained. The training provided little opportunity to impart an understanding of the importance of a 'development perspective'. There is considerable anecdotal evidence of Western Australian children being diagnosed and prescribed by a paediatrician after a fifteen-minute (and sometimes even shorter) consultation. Halasz pointed to reduced time for patient care and believed that even fifty to sixty minutes were inadequate to assess the development of a child's symptoms.

The 2004 parliamentary inquiry into ADHD supported Halasz's view. It found that the shortage in Perth of appropriately trained child psychiatrists to perform time-intensive diagnoses and treatments left a vacuum filled by a relatively small number of inadequately trained paediatricians who diagnosed and prescribed quickly. The inquiry was convinced by the evidence that seeing a paediatrician as opposed to a mental health professional (i.e. a psychiatrist) was a 'risk factor in the use of stimulant medication'.[15]

Perth's Adult Prescribing Rates Continue to Rise

Although rates for children have fallen, those for adults have not. When a full year's data first became available from the stimulants monitoring regime it revealed that in 2005 there were 6756 adults who received stimulants.[16] By 2008 this number had risen to 7139, with adults in the prosperous Oceanic Health District nearly twice as likely as other metropolitan Perth adults to have received a script.[17] This 6 per cent growth in adult numbers is not surprising given the number of former child patients who are now young adults and the considerable effort put into marketing adult ADHD. How many of these adult patients are genuinely seeking help and how many are after a cheap source of amphetamines is impossible to know.

The 1990s: A Decade of WA State Government Policy Failure

Concerns about Western Australian rates of prescription and the diagnostic practices of some unnamed Perth paediatricians first emerged in the mid 1990s.[18] In 1995 the Court Liberal state government set up the Technical Working Party on Attention Deficit Disorder 'to report to government on the incidence of ADHD in Western Australia and to seek expert opinion on the appropriate diagnosis and treatment for the condition'.[19] *The Report of the Technical Working Party on Attention Deficit Disorder to the Cabinet Sub-Committee* highlighted that, in 1994, Western Australian child prescription rates were about two and a half times the national average, and that there had been a massive (forty-three-fold) growth in the prescription of dexamphetamine to five- to fourteen-year-olds between 1989 and 1994.[20]

The *Report of the Technical Working Party* identified two ADHD hotspots: one in Perth's affluent western suburbs where I taught from 1995 to 2000, and the other in Perth's economically disadvantaged south-east corridor, which I first represented when I entered parliament from 2001 to 2005. It concluded this patchy geographical distribution was probably 'more reflective of the prescribing patterns of paediatricians servicing the various areas than it is of social or other factors'.[21] To address this inconsistency in prescribing rates it recommended 'random audits into the use of block authorisations, and that paediatricians and psychiatrists found to be failing to abide by the appropriate criteria have their block authorisation capacity removed'.[22]

Block authorisation exempted frequently prescribing clinicians from the requirement to get authorisation for each individual prescription. In effect, it meant that frequent prescribers were the least accountable. In contrast, a clinician who prescribed infrequently, as a last resort, was accountable for every individual script. Presumably the rationale for the policy of 'block authorisation' was the assumption that those who prescribed frequently were considered to be 'familiar with the guidelines for prescribing stimulants'.[23] This seems completely irrational – why wouldn't the heaviest prescribers have been the most accountable?

In response to the Working Party recommendations the Western Australian Stimulants Committee was established by the Western Australian Department of Health in 1997. The Stimulants Committee was supposed to monitor the prescription of psychostimulants to ensure appropriate prescribing. The

Committee included some of Perth's heaviest prescribers, who themselves had block authorisation, and were therefore exempt from oversight. Not surprisingly, the recommended audits of block authorisation never happened.

Drs Trevor Parry and Ken Whiting were members of the Stimulants Committee from its inception in 1997 until it was abolished in 2003. Both benefited from the exemption from accountability provided by block authorisation.[24] Stimulants Committee meeting minutes from 20 February 2002 recorded:

> As there were a number of applications outside the mg/kg range, Dr Oleh Kay, enquired if it would be possible to have en-bloc authorisation for doses outside the mg/kg[25]...Dr Whiting said he would be pleased to be exempt in this case and he advised that Dr Parry would be also...Dr Harris advised that the Department could not be put in a position where members of the Committee had en-bloc authorisation to prescribe outside the mg/kg range, as this would understandably be seen to be bias.[26]

Drs Whiting and Parry were the 'policemen' who were supposed to be ensuring the safe and responsible prescription of amphetamines in Western Australia. According to Dr Whiting they were happy to extend their personal accountability exemptions to allow them to prescribe outside the manufacturers' prescribing guidelines. Dr Linda Harris at least deserves credit for pointing out the obvious conflict of interest.

Other Stimulants Committee minutes obtained through Freedom of Information (FOI) revealed that the Committee took a softly-softly approach to the most reckless prescribers, even when their prescribing resulted in children being hospitalised. The names of the doctors with the questionable prescribing practices were not disclosed in the FOI documents.

The minutes refer to an unnamed doctor (Dr Z) whose child patient was hospitalised because of 'abnormal limb movements, slurred speech and unusual behaviour' after being prescribed Ritalin at an extraordinarily high dose in combination with 'several' other drugs. The 6mg/kg dose was potentially fatal and many multiples of the recommended dosage range. While Dr Z had block authorisation, he still needed to apply for special authority to prescribe at that level – therefore his actions were illegal. The Stimulants Committee took no formal action save for organising a meeting with Dr Z which was 'felt to be fruitful'. Perhaps the most revealing comment minuted was 'that although the stimulant dose was high these were inherently safe drugs and yet there was no prescribing restrictions of other far more dangerous drugs'. If the committee was not prepared to act after a prescribed overdose of amphetamine saw a child hospitalised to detox then they probably never would (and they never did).[27]

In 1999 there were concerns about a Dr H and 'the large numbers of applications outside the guidelines that he had submitted...not only at the large doses but also at the low weights and young ages of the patients', which prompted an advisory meeting between members of the Stimulants Committee and Dr H. At the meeting Dr H 'acknowledged that some of his patients were on up to 25 tablets daily but they seemed to be doing well...[and]...he was aware of the possible problem of patients selling tablets'. While the Stimulants Committee sent an advisory letter and organised two 'fruitful' meetings, it took no decisive action. This did not significantly change Dr H's prescribing practices. While they did discuss the prospect of curtailing his block authorisation capacity and making him accountable for every script (as is now required of all prescribers), change only occurred when Dr H left the state.[28]

The Committee was not even prepared to take action against illegal prescribers. Dr X, who was neither a paediatrician nor a psychiatrist and was therefore not able to initiate a patient on stimulants, prescribed a patient with dexamphetamine even though it was 'contraindicated in this patient' as he had 'psychotic symptoms with emerging schizophrenia'. The committee considered two options: recommending to the Western Australian Health Department that 'action be taken against Dr X as it is illegal what he has allegedly done', or that the Department write to Dr X advising him not to 'prescribe dexamphetamine or supply it without authorisation from the Commissioner of Health'. The committee initially decided on the second softer option and then failed to follow through. The draft letter was never sent but 'retained on file and if another allegation comes forward then the Department will have more weight in which to write to him'. [29]

Further minutes disclose the Committee's enthusiasm for fewer restrictions on prescribing. The Committee discussed the option of dropping 'the age for stimulant prescribing from 4 years of age down to 3 years of age', with 'members agreed that earlier intervention is the best way'.[30] The Committee also approved two applications that dexamphetamine be used outside guidelines during pregnancy. Committee members, notably Dr Trevor Parry, argued that for paediatricians, 'provided they [did] not initiate treatment for [people] over 18 years of age, there should be the freedom for continuity of care and [this] should not be seen as a problem'.[31]

The Stimulants Committee gave the appearance of requiring accountability of prescribers. However, it was dominated by prescribers with an enormous professional investment in the validity of ADHD, and stimulants as a safe and effective treatment. It was another example of a government delegating concerns about ADHD prescription practices to those with a vested self-interest. While the Stimulants Committee, including Drs Whiting and Parry, failed to restrict the activities of Drs Z, H and X, who was overseeing the prescribing practices of Drs Whiting, Parry and others who enjoyed the freedom of block authorisation?

Between 1997 and 2000 along with instituting the Stimulants Committee, other isolated and ineffective efforts to rein in ADHD prescribing rates took place. In September 1999 the Western Australian Department of Mental Health convened a three-day symposium to address concerns 'about the number of WA children diagnosed with attention deficit disorder and the use of amphetamine-like medication to treat them'.[32] The Department invited 'international experts' including Professor Larry Greenhill of New York's Columbia University. Professor Greenhill is on the payroll of fifteen pharmaceutical companies and, typical of ADHD 'experts', is a fervent and motivated advocate of ADHD prescribing. (See chapter 5.) Predictably the symposium did nothing to inhibit burgeoning prescribing rates.

Although the majority of Western Australian doctors believed that dexamphetamine was over-prescribed this was a silent majority.[33] Heavy prescribers may not have enjoyed the overwhelming support of their colleagues, but with all too few exceptions they did not suffer their criticism either. One of the most frustrating aspects of my own advocacy regarding ADHD has been the number of Perth doctors who have privately congratulated me. Initially I found their covert encouragement gratifying; however, over time I have become frustrated at their unwillingness to express their views publicly. This reluctance to get involved has meant self-regulation by the cliquey Western Australian medical fraternity has failed spectacularly.

The Turning Point: The Abolition of Block Authorisation

Concerns about 1994 prescribing rates, when less than 1 per cent of children were on stimulants, first led to suggestions to curtail block authorisation.[34] Seven years later in 2001, when I was elected as the Member for Roleystone as part of the new Gallop Labor government, the total number of PBS-subsidised dexamphetamine scripts had increased sixfold.[35]

I raised the issue of block authorisation in my inaugural speech stating, 'the problem of block authorisation continues. I believe making doctors accountable on a case-by-case basis for the prescription of stimulant medication is essential to dealing with the problem of over prescription'.[36] The change of govern-ment, my election and the appointment of the Honourable Bob Kucera as health minister, provided the opportunity for the direction of policy to be reversed. Bob Kucera, a former senior policeman has seen the problems caused by the diversion of amphetamines prescribed for ADHD.

In 2002 the report *Attentional Problems in Children and Young People* was published by the Western Australian Mental Health Division. An earlier draft of the report promoted ADHD. It emphasised developing a tiered approach, with teachers and childcare workers spotting potential ADHD children and referring them up the chain for diagnosis by specialist clinicians. The draft report was, with my input, radically altered by Minister Kucera's office. The final draft abandoned the 'tiered spotters' approach and recommended the abolition of block authorisation as well as the establishment of multidisciplinary clinics to diagnose and treat children with behavioural and learning problems. Minister Kucera announced the decision to end block authorisation in December 2002 and the practice was stopped in August 2003. The Stimulants Committee was replaced by the Stimulants Panel and had a significantly different membership. After block authorisation was abolished all authorised prescribers were equally accountable for each prescription.[37]

Minister Kucera's and my own enthusiasm for the end of block authorisation and for the new accountability measures was not shared by everyone. The then president of the Western Australian branch of the Australian Medical Association Dr Bernard Pearn-Rowe said:

> Families should have no doubt that the Health Minister is trying to take away the ability of a doctor to make clinical decisions in consultation with parents...I hope the Minister will tell individual parents that his policy is responsible for the refusal of treatment, even when recommended as appropriate by a qualified medical practitioner.[38]

Regardless of Dr Pearn-Rowe's criticisms, the abolition of block authorisation was followed by a massive decrease in the estimate of the number of children on stimulants from 18,000 in 2000 to less than 6000 in 2008. Perth is the world's only ADHD hot spot to have seen such a dramatic downturn in prescribing rates for children.

Greater Detail on WA Child ADHD Prescribing Rates

Prior to the abolition of block authorisation and the introduction of the new stimulants monitoring system, information about ADHD prescribing rates was limited to total script numbers provided through the PBS. It was difficult to know the numbers of children and adults who were on ADHD medications or the doses they received. As previously stated the Western Australian Department of Health estimated there were 20,648 people on ADHD stimulants in WA in 2000.[39] Based on available information from NSW, it was estimated between 85 per cent (17,551) and 90 per cent (18,583) were children (0–17). By 2005 the number of children on ADHD stimulants had fallen dramatically to 8057, a fall of approximately 55 per cent.[40] Even if the estimates of children as a proportion of the ADHD cohort was an overestimate and the proportion of the ADHD cohort in 2000 was only 70 per cent (14,597) this represents a fall in child ADHD prescribing rates of over 44 per cent. Subsequent to the initial fall, child-prescribing rates have continued to decline, with the number of children prescribed stimulants in 2008 totalling 5666.[41] Using the Health Department's official estimate this represents over 12,000 fewer children on ADHD stimulants or a fall of nearly 70 per cent. Using the more conservative estimate, it still means nearly 9000 fewer children on ADHD stimulants, or a fall of over 60 per cent.

The first annual report of the stimulants monitoring regime revealed a single Perth paediatrician was responsible for prescribing to 2077 children in the 17 months from August 2003 to December 2004. This was 21.5 per cent of all ADHD child patients prescribed in WA over that period.[42] This is clearly an absurd number for a single practitioner who must have been doing little more than meeting, diagnosing, prescribing and forgetting. However, Perth's heaviest prescriber was no lone ranger. Over the same seventeen-month period in WA, fifteen of the 172 authorised prescribers were responsible for prescribing to over 7300 (nearly half) patients who received stimulants.

These figures were collected after the tighter accountability measures were put in place, and there is no way of knowing how many patients were prescribed by individual clinicians before the spotlight was put on them.

Conclusion: Where to from Here?

I have never heard it argued that current diagnosing and prescribing rates for ADHD are appropriate. There are three schools of thought on ADHD and all are critical of these rates. The ADHD industry's extreme position, which while it is a minority view has dominated clinical practice, is that ADHD is an under-diagnosed, under-medicated, inherited, biochemical imbalance in the brain that is best treated with 'safe, 'effective' medication. At the other end of the spectrum are powerful and persuasive arguments that ADHD is a total fraud and not a valid psychiatric diagnosis. The middle view is that ADHD is frequently misdiagnosed and over-prescribed. Opinion leaders who are worried about the damage done by ADHD labelling and drugging often express concerns about misdiagnosis and over-prescription. In my maiden parliamentary speech given in May 2001 I said, 'I now have grave concerns that ADD

misdiagnosis and the resultant over-prescription of amphetamines is a threat to the health and happiness of many Western
Australian children.'[1]

Implicit in my statement is that ADHD is a legitimate diag-
nosable disorder or disease and that some children with ADHD
should take amphetamines. The attraction of this middle position for those expressing a public view, particularly politicians,
is that showing concern, but taking the middle ground, appears
and feels responsible and reasonable. It is less confronting to say
that a minority of practitioners overdo diagnosis and prescription than it is to assert that the psychiatric profession and major
medical associations and government health agencies have got it
completely wrong and that ADHD is a fraud. Expediency aside,
questions remain. When I said ADHD was misdiagnosed and
over-medicated, was I right to accept implicitly the validity of
a lower level of ADHD medicating? Is ADHD a legitimate disorder or disease and, if so, are amphetamines good for children
with ADHD?

Having been so deeply immersed in the detail of the debate
I have changed my 2001 position. In 2006 I told the WA state
Parliament:

> I did argue that ADHD is over-diagnosed and over-
> prescribed. I now say ADHD is a fraud – this is how
> my position has changed, not because kids do not have
> real things going on in their lives, but simply because
> the bar for diagnosing the condition is far too low.[2]

The concept that ADHD is a biochemical brain imbalance
causing dysfunctional inattentive and/or impulsive behaviour is

at best an unproven hypothesis. However, when this unproven hypothesis is assumed to be fact and used as the rationale for drugging children with amphetamines, it constitutes a dangerous fraud.

ADHD is a fraud because virtually any child could be diagnosed. ADHD is a fraud because the drug company sponsored pseudo-science that has been used to justify the wholesale drugging of children fails to adhere to the basic rules of good science. ADHD is a fraud because it fails the commonsense test. The whole fraud hangs on the unsupported assumption of a biochemical brain imbalance and the generalised temporary behaviour-altering qualities of low-dose amphetamines. Stimulant medication acts in precisely the way it is intended to. It stimulates. This does not mean that it is treating a problem or fixing a chemical imbalance. Stimulants are simply acting as temporary behaviour modifiers, with compelling evidence of long-term educational disadvantage and cardiovascular damage.

Some of the strongest critics of current ADHD diagnosing and prescribing practices are clinicians who very occasionally prescribe for a condition they describe as 'true ADHD'. They hold the middle view that 'true ADHD' is a real but very rare condition. They believe that a very small number of children can benefit from medication when its dose is low and controlled, and it is used as a short-term, monitored intervention. Clinicians holding and prescribing in line with this view do not typically use the American Psychiatric Association's DSM-IV as the working diagnostic criteria. They use the World Health Organization's more narrowly defined ICD-10 diagnostic criteria, even then adding rigour and only prescribing to a small number of children diagnosed with extreme hyperkinetic disorder. These responsible clinicians argue that the bar for diagnosing ADHD is too low, and criticise DSM-IV and to a lesser extent ICD-10. Instead of completely rejecting the term ADHD, however, they talk about 'true ADHD' without ever defining it. The psychiatric profession has a duty to define in clear unequivocal terms what they mean when they talk about 'true ADHD'. A few clinicians have demonstrated that in the absence of a meaningful definition, they have the ability to make judgment calls. They talk responsibly and prescribe reluctantly. Experience tells us, however, that too many clinicians talk responsibly, and prescribe recklessly.

Psychiatry's history of lobotomies, deep sleep therapy, eugenics and now pharmaceutical psychiatry has repeatedly taught us that a significant and dangerous minority within the profession cannot be trusted to exercise this discretion judiciously. Furthermore, extending this discretion to paediatricians and general practitioners who lack full psychiatric training and have a demonstrated propensity for dumbed down checklist psychiatry is even more problematic. The onus falls on the medical profession and governments to ensure that only those appropriately trained in holistic psychiatry can practise psychiatry. Most importantly the onus falls on the psychiatric profession to act like a science-based profession. It must come up with a reliable scientific diagnosis based on aetiology and not on observations that children are exhibiting childish behaviours like playing too loudly and not waiting their turn. If the psychiatric profession cannot do that then it must abandon the concept of ADHD or abandon its claims to be a profession.

So far the medical profession in general, and psychiatry in particular, have failed to self-regulate. With a few notable exceptions they have turned a blind eye to rogue prescribers and allowed children to suffer. Politicians and governments have done no better. With evidence emerging of sloppy diagnostic practices, long-term harm and commercially corrupted pro-drug research, it is perhaps time for the legal profession to step in where the medical profession and government have failed. Lawyers applying the 'tort of negligence' may provide better protection of children's rights than the Hippocratic obligation for doctors to 'first do no harm'.

The ADHD epidemic did not happen by accident. It is a manufactured epidemic where the scientific process has been corrupted by drug company profits. Many parents have been scared into drugging their child and seduced by the temporary behaviour-altering effects of amphetamines. Like the fabled adulation of the emperor's new clothes, the growth of and enthusiasm for ADHD ignores the blindingly obvious. In the minds of the medical profession, educators, politicians and policy makers, ADHD has got so big it must be real. But, like the emperor's new clothes, ADHD has no substance. If ADHD were a genetically determined biochemical imbalance then medicating to balance the brain's biochemistry would perhaps be a logical and responsible treatment. But ADHD is no more than an unsupported theory. Drugging millions of children worldwide with amphetamines on the basis that poorly defined behavioural evidence is proof of a biochemical imbalance is a massive abuse of children's rights. This madness must end.

Appendix 1

Strattera's Sad Short Story
(Warning – it may make you want to kill yourself)

Strattera is Eli Lilly's brand name for atomoxetine hydrochloride, a noradrenaline reuptake inhibitor. Strattera's legitimate marketing edge is that unlike dexamphetamine and methylphenidate, it is not amphetamine based and therefore has the advantage of being non-addictive and unsuitable for illicit use. It was first trialled in 1982 as an antidepressant branded Tomoxetine but was found to be ineffective.[1] Eli Lilly refused a request to release results of trials of Tomoxetine as an antidepressant stating:

> ...it is important to note that the population in these trials is different from the population in which atomoxetine hydrochloride is approved for use by the TGA in Australia. As a result, the relevance of the trials for current clinical practice is significantly diminished.[2]

Given Strattera's now established propensity to cause suicidal ideation, it is obvious why it was unsuitable as an antidepressant. Eli Lilly was determined not to waste its investment in product development and re-branded Tomoxetine as Strattera, a revolutionary non-stimulant ADHD drug. In 2002 the US FDA approved Strattera for the treatment of ADHD. It was approved in Australia in early 2004.

Eli Lilly achieved approval of Strattera in the standard way. That is, Eli Lilly funded the research, set the parameters, controlled the dissemination of the results and handpicked and paid the researchers. I randomly chose one of the studies that supported Eli Lilly's initial application for approval to analyse its independence. The study 'Atomoxetine in the Treatment of Children and Adolescents with Attention-Deficit/ Hyperactivity Disorder: A Randomized, Placebo-Controlled, Dose-Response Study' was published in 2001.[3] All eighteen authors had pre-existing financial ties to Eli Lilly, with five being shareholders and/or employees. The study was not blind rated. Many of the raters were paid by Eli Lilly and the most neutral potential raters, teachers, in the most relevant setting, schools, were excluded from the study.

> **Summary of 'Atomoxetine in the Treatment of Children and Adolescents With Attention-Deficit/Hyperactivity Disorder: A Randomized, Placebo-Controlled, Dose-Response Study'**
> The study is attributed to eighteen authors, David Michelson, Douglas Faries, PhD; Joachim Wernicke, MD, PhD, Douglas Kelsey, MD, PhD, Katherine Kendrick, BS, F. Randy Sallee, MD, PhD, Thomas Spencer, MD and eleven members (mostly MDs) of the Atomoxetine ADHD Study Group. Drs Sallee and Spencer (see chapter 5) and all eleven members of the study group

'have acted as paid consultants and/or investigators for studies sponsored by Eli Lilly and Company'.[4] The other five individually identified authors 'Drs Michelson, Faries, Wernicke, and Kelsey and Ms Kendrick are employees and shareholders of Eli Lilly and Company'.[5]

The rationale for the study was that 'Several reports have provided evidence that atomoxetine is superior to placebo in reducing symptoms of ADHD in children and adults. However, the relative efficacy and the relative safety and tolerability of different doses have not been assessed.' Given that Eli Lilly funded the study, and all eighteen authors had financial ties to the company, it is hardly surprising that the results supported the use of Strattera:

> The data reported here provide additional evidence
> of the efficacy and safety of atomoxetine in older
> children and adolescents with ADHD and that
> successful treatment with atomoxetine is associated
> with both symptomatic and functional improvement.[6]

The study assessed ADHD symptoms, affective symptoms, and social and family functioning using parent and investigator rating scales. It included 297 eight- to eighteen-year-olds diagnosed with ADHD and concluded: 'Social and family functioning also were improved in the atomoxetine groups compared with placebo with statistically significant improvements in measures of children's ability to meet psychosocial role expectations and parental impact.'[7] There was an obvious bias in that one source of ratings, the investigators, received payment from Eli Lilly. Additionally, as the study was not blinded and parents knew whether the child was medicated or un-medicated, parent ratings must be viewed with suspicion. Even if parents noticed children were more compliant, this benefit is external to the child. The children were not asked how the medication affected them.

Hype

Among pharmaceutical companies Eli Lilly has a well-earned reputation as one of the most aggressive marketers. Its entry into the ADHD market was well resourced and dogmatic. Eli Lilly's website on Strattera contained a section entitled 'What Is ADHD?' It stated, 'Attention-Deficit/Hyperactivity Disorder is a neurological condition related, in part, to the brain's chemistry and anatomy' which 'manifests itself as a persistent pattern of inattention and/or hyperactivity-impulsivity' and that 'While some children outgrow ADHD, about 60 per cent continue to have symptoms into adulthood.'[8] It presents the hypothesis that the aetiology is 'neurological', related to 'brain chemistry and anatomy', and that in most cases ADHD is a life-long condition, as if it were a certainty.

In the US Eli Lilly marketed Strattera for adult ADHD in a way that blurs the lines between the stresses of modern life and disease. An advertisement for Strattera in the *US News & World Report* reads:

> Distracted? Disorganized? Frustrated? Modern Life or Adult ADD? Many adults have been living with Adult attention deficit disorder and don't recognize it. Why? because its symptoms are often mistaken for stressful life.[9]

Eli Lilly has also made a habit of making unsubstantiated claims about Strattera. In June 2005, exaggerated claims in an American TV advertisement attracted the ire of the Food and Drug Administration, which issued a warning letter stating: 'The TV ad is false or misleading because it inadequately communicates the indication for Strattera and minimizes the risks associated with Strattera.'[10]

In Australia Eli Lilly publicised Strattera's non-addictive properties in an environment of growing concern about the safety of stimulants, and their illicit use. In Western Australia Strattera was promoted through a very favourable article 'Drug to cut schoolyard trade' in the *West Australian* newspaper on 16 April 2004:

> A new non-stimulant drug to treat attention deficit hyperactivity disorder released in Australia this week could help cut the school playground trade in 'kiddy speed', a Perth paediatrician has claimed. Ken Whiting said atomoxetine hydrochloride, sold as Strattera, was a once-daily drug which did not contain the stimulants amphetamine or methylphenidate. Excluding stimulants also eliminated the possibility of addiction. Substance abuse is known to be higher in people with ADHD, although that risk can be reduced by up to 50 per cent with treatment. WA support group The Learning and Attentional Disorders Society (LADS) of WA (spokeswoman Michelle Toner) said families would welcome new, clinically proved options for better ADHD management.[11]

> *Note:* LADS has received support from Eli Lilly and Dr Ken Whiting was a key member of LADS.

The following day another favourable article entitled 'Aid for new ADHD drug sought' appeared in the *West Australian* lobbying for Strattera to be subsidised via the Pharmaceutical

Benefits Scheme. The article quoted Western Australian Secondary School Executives' Association president Ray Maher as saying 'the drug could be a boon to schools and particularly principals ultimately responsible for ensuring the security and correct administration of dexamphetamines – sometimes referred to as kiddie speed'.[12]

At the same time more articles promoting Strattera's non-addictive advantage appeared in other Australian newspapers. Page 3 of the Brisbane *Courier Mail* carried an article titled 'New drug combats child addiction fears'. It quoted Dr Michael McDowell, a developmental pediatrician from the Child Development Network at Brisbane's Mater Hospital who conducted the Australian clinical trials of Strattera, as saying: 'The fear parents have of amphetamines...is the possibility of addiction and abuse, whereas this current medication doesn't come with that risk.'[13] Page 3 of the *Sydney Morning Herald* carried an article titled 'Milder new drug hailed for attention disorder'. It also quoted McDowell:

> There is no risk they will take too much for a psychological high...there's no risk they will sell it on to other children in the playground because it can't be taken as a recreational drug. But it does have similar side effects to the other drugs including abdominal pain, decreased appetite, increased blood pressure and vomiting. There are side effects, but overall they're milder and I suspect the likelihood that parents would stop the medication because of side effects is less than existing medications.[14]

Comments like McDowell's, and the fact that Strattera was non-addictive made it seem a safer option than stimulants. Even I thought it deserved consideration and so in December 2003 I visited Eli Lilly's Australian headquarters in Sydney. I later told the WA Parliament:

> I visited Eli Lilly's office in Sydney to hear its Strattera pitch. I had an open mind and was hoping for a harmless alternative to dexamphetamine and Ritalin; however, I was disturbed to encounter the reluctance of Lilly's three representatives to answer one very simple, straightforward question: what are the side effects or dangers of Strattera? I became suspicious as a result of that reluctance, and it did not take a long time to have my suspicions confirmed.[15]

Reality

Despite Eli Lilly's hype and Dr McDowell's claims of a milder ADHD drug, concerns emerged about its safety soon after Strattera came on the market. On 17 December 2004 the US FDA issued a talk paper, 'New Warning for Strattera', which stated:

> The drug's labeling is being updated with a bolded warning about the potential for severe liver injury in patients taking Strattera. The label warns that severe liver injury can progress to liver failure in a small percentage of patients. It cautions clinicians to discontinue the drug in patients who develop jaundice or

laboratory evidence of liver injury. It also notes that the actual number of cases of severe liver injury from the drug is not known because of under-reporting.[16]

Soon after the FDA warning, the Australian Therapeutic Goods Administration altered the Consumer Medicine Information for Strattera, but made no public announcement.

Less than a year after the information about potentially fatal liver damage came to light and less than two years after Strattera came on to the market, even more disturbing information emerged. On 29 September 2005 the FDA issued a public health advisory announcing they had put the highest possible black box warning on Strattera for suicidal ideation:

> Strattera increases the risk of suicidal thinking in children and adolescents with ADHD. Patients who are started on therapy should be observed closely for clinical worsening, suicidal thinking or behaviours, or unusual changes in behaviour. Families and caregivers should be advised to closely observe the patient and to communicate changes or concerning behaviours with the prescriber.[17]

This health advisory was well publicised in the US and attracted considerable media attention. As well as publicising the warning, the FDA insisted that specific information about these dangers be provided to consumers with every new prescription of Strattera.[18] In contrast the TGA made little effort to publicise this disturbing information. While six months later (on 19 March 2006) they did put a boxed warning for suicidal ideation on the product information made available to pre-scribers, they did not issue a press release to ensure parents were informed. The decision about whether to inform parents and/or patients for suicidality was left with individual prescribers. Perth paediatrician Dr Ken Whiting trusted Eli Lilly to be the key information provider stating, 'the drug company is trying to make practitioners aware of it so that we can watch patients and ensure there's no problems. It's important that patients don't stop taking the drug suddenly but see their doctor.'[19] The TGA did not alert Australian media about the warnings or any subsequent adverse event reports of suicidal behaviour.

It wasn't until November 2006, when I became aware of the warnings and reports and raised the issue of the TGA's extremely low-key response to the WA Parliament, that they got significant media coverage.[20] I stated:

Although it [the TGA] put a black-box warning of suicide on Strattera on 19 March 2006, it did almost nothing to inform the public of this. Even the term 'black-box warning' is extremely misleading. Until recently, I mistakenly assumed that it was a promi-nent warning written in black on the outside of drug packaging. However, I was mistaken. In reality, it is the warning on the product information sheet that is available only to doctors, not patients or parents. Apart from the inadequate, hard-to-find, softly worded information in consumer medicine information, there is no mechanism for ensuring that parents and patients are informed. The TGA had no excuse for its half-baked response...The TGA has done almost nothing to warn parents that Strattera could cause their children's liver to fail or cause their children to want to kill themselves.[21]

When my comments and the information about adverse events were eventually reported, Eli Lilly issued a press release:

> Eli Lilly stands by the safety profile of Strattera. It is an important treatment option for people diagnosed with ADHD. We also stand by the rigorous processes put into place by the TGA to ensure patient safety. As Mr Whitely pointed out, following the emergence of new safety-related data, we reported it immediately to the TGA and action was undertaken to update public safety information. Eli Lilly worked closely with the TGA to actively inform prescribing specialists, GPs and pharmacists of the new precautions in the product information to ensure they are able to monitor patients accordingly. All relevant ADHD patient support groups were informed at the time of the Product Information update. An update was posted on the Eli Lilly website.[22]

Eli Lilly's assurance that all relevant ADHD patient support groups were informed is revealing. In Western Australia LADS, who Eli Lilly supports and which promotes its products, was informed. The group DFADS (Drug Free Attention Difficulties Support), which I founded, which promotes drug free approaches for children with attentional difficulties, was not.[23] At no point did Eli Lilly refute the facts contained in my parliamentary speech. Their press release added little except to emphasise how 'Eli Lilly worked closely with the TGA'. Regulators like the TGA should make drug companies, who produce products that make children want to kill themselves very uncomfortable. Eli Lilly were obviously very comfortable as they praised the 'rigorous process put in place by the TGA'.

From 2004, when Strattera first came on to the market, until 7 May 2009, there were eighty-seven voluntary adverse event reports, including thirty-nine of suicidality.[24] With Ritalin and dexamphetamine, it is impossible to know the true number of actual events, as the voluntary nature of the reporting system means only a fraction of the actual incidents gets reported.[25]

A Sample from the Adverse Drug Reactions Committee (ADRAC) adverse event reports for Atomoxetine Hydrochloride (Strattera)

- seven-year-old girl who tried to kill herself and 'became very agitated while travelling in the family car and had explosive mood swings. She said that she intended to open the door and get out of the car, and she tried to open the car door';
- seven-year-old boy who experienced 'suicidal ideation and mood changes' and suffered from 'increased aggression' and 'threats to self with knife, picking his skin, poking self with knife';
- eight-year-old boy who 'hit his head against a wall' and had 'thoughts of suicide – stating that he wants to kill himself';
- nine-year-old boy who expressed 'suicidal ideation',

'aggression' and 'self harm' and made 'drawings of him hanging upside down from tree, in (the) ocean';

- nine-year-old boy who slammed 'his head against walls, had extreme mood swings, violent outbursts' and was 'always angry, depressed or sad and said he wanted to kill himself';
- ten-year-old-boy who was psychotic and experienced auditory hallucinations, including 'hearing voices in his head to kill his sister';
- ten-year-old boy who 'experienced nausea, then became acutely depressed, aggressive and had suicidal thoughts';
- eleven-year-old boy who 'attempted suicide' and who experienced 'headache(s), stomach cramps, muscle rigidity and poor concentration';
- twelve-year-old girl who experienced 'anorexia, weight loss, fidgeting and compulsive behaviour that included ripping out fingernails and toenails, picking and cutting clothing, and anger outbursts';
- thirteen-year-old boy who 'experienced chest pains and hostile and aggressive behaviour, but the problems immediately disappeared with the cessation of Strattera'.

Curtin University's Strattera Study

Since Strattera's entry into the market Eli Lilly and Australian taxpayers have funded further research to establish the safety and efficacy of use by children and adolescents.

In 2004 Associate Professor Heather Jenkins, a Western Australian psychologist from Curtin University's Faculty of Education, led a study comparing Strattera to dexamphetamine as a treatment for children diagnosed with ADHD. She voluntarily gave evidence to the 2004 Western Australian parliamentary inquiry into ADHD. The following is an excerpt from an exchange with Associate Professor Jenkins in which Jenkins 'corrects' me for stating dexamphetamine is addictive:

Mr M. P. Whitely: I am interested in hearing a little bit about the study on the use of Strattera because I have visited Eli Lilly Australia in Sydney. I must say that it was difficult to get information, but one of the side effects seemed quite similar to those of dexamphetamine and Ritalin. However, Eli Lilly said that one of the benefits was that Strattera had less addictive properties (than dexamphetamine) so there were fewer black market issues than there were previously. Can you tell me a little bit about the study, what it is trying to achieve and Eli Lilly's involvement in it? One of the criticisms we have continually heard is that much of the research is funded by drug companies that obviously have a vested interest. It is therefore an obvious question that needs to be asked. What is Eli Lilly's involvement in the study, is it funding it, what control does it have over it, and how is it conducted?

A/Prof H. Jenkins: First, dexamphetamine is not addictive, if I might correct your earlier comment.

Mr M. P. Whitely: Okay. Let us talk about atomoxetine [Strattera].

A/Prof H. Jenkins: I object to statements being made that in my opinion are incorrect.

THE DEPUTY CHAIRMAN: What we are trying to do is to get your opinion rather than argue the case. If the witness could just answer the question.

MR M. P. WHITELY: GlaxoSmithKline Australia thinks it is addictive. It is the manufacturer (of dexamphetamine). Anyway, we will not go into that.

THE DEPUTY CHAIRMAN: We want to draw out your opinion on these matters. We can argue the case later in committee. If we could have your opinion.

A/PROF H. JENKINS: The study is an independently initiated trial. I am an independent investigator. Eli Lilly has signed all forms that are issued by Curtin University. Curtin University owns the intellectual property of all outcomes. They will be published in peer-reviewed scholarly journals. Eli Lilly's involvement is necessary because it will supply the Strattera. It will not supply the dexamphetamine. There is a control group for dexamphetamine and a control group for atomoxetine. I cannot obtain atomoxetine other than through Eli Lilly. At the present time I am going through all the approval procedures for Eli Lilly to approve this study and issue the atomoxetine. Other than that, Eli Lilly has funded me $15,000 a year for three years. It has handed over a cheque for the first $30,000. It has asked for no accountability whatsoever. It has not influenced me in any way; it has not influenced my presentations at conferences, my publications or any other aspects of my work. The study will also have to meet all the National Health and Medical Research Council ethical guidelines.[26]

Associate Professor Jenkins's aggressive ignorance of the addictive nature of dexamphetamine concerned me. Given that the control in her study was dexamphetamine and not a placebo, I considered it was her responsibility to understand the risks of administering the drug. I did not trust her to fully inform parents of the suicidality associated with Strattera, or her claims of independence from Eli Lilly. Consequently, I requested through Freedom of Information, documents from Associate Professor Jenkins's study, in order to find out three specific things:

1. How much funding had been provided by Eli Lilly and did they exert any influence on its conduct?

2. What had the Curtin University ethics committee been told about the possible adverse side effects of Strattera, particularly in relation to suicidal ideation?

3. What had parents been told about those possible same side effects?

Curtin University refused to provide the requested documents explaining that:

> In the view of the University there is public confidence in research in Universities and it would not be in the public interest to compromise research by making public procedures and deliberations and research details that are accepted generally as being confidential.[27]

I considered that 'public confidence in research in Universities' could and should only be maintained if the research was robust, ethical and independent of commercial influence. Fifteen months later, after an appeal to the Western Australian Freedom of Information Commissioner, which the university contested, the Commissioner found in my favour and I was provided with all the documentation I requested.

In addition to her assurance to the parliamentary inquiry that the study was independent of Eli Lilly's influence, Associate Professor Jenkins claimed in a statement to parents of children in the study that:

> Eli Lilly has signed an agreement with Curtin University of Technology that confirms that the university investigators are completely independent of their company. This means that Eli Lilly Australia has not influenced the design of the study.[28]

However, 'the FOI documents show that a drug company employee was paid to work on the study as an investigator, who would contribute to the overall conduct of the study through advice on design and implementation'.[29] An email from Eli Lilly's director of corporate affairs and health economics to Associate Professor Jenkins in 2002, sent during the set-up phase of the project, stated:

> We (Eli Lilly) would like the opportunity for our clinical research physician to look at the proposed protocol in more depth. We have some initial thoughts regarding a couple of additional instruments that may be worth including.[30]

Eli Lilly had 'contributed $145,000 in cash and in-kind support to the trial. The trial also received a $500,000 grant from taxpayers via the Australian Research Council.'[31] Clearly Eli

Lilly, in contravention of Associate Professor Jenkins's assurance to parents, was seeking to influence the design of the study.

Just as she had erred with her statement about dexamphetamine being non-addictive, Jenkins completely misunderstood the risks associated with Strattera. She informed Curtin's Human Research Ethics Committee in June 2006 that the US Food and Drug Administration had revoked a black box warning about the increased risk of suicidal thoughts; she cited an article which had appeared in the US medical journal *Pediatric News*:

> Since the study has been approved, there [have] been some publications related to the rare occurrence of suicidal ideation in some patients who were taking Strattera. This initially led to a black-box warning from the FDA, which was subsequently revoked following further investigations.[32]

This was wrong. The FDA black box warning had been in place for eight months (and the TGA's for two months) at the time Jenkins advised the committee it had been lifted and the article she cited said so.[33]

It is unclear if parents were ever fully informed about the risks of Strattera:

> [a] document provided by the university to parents of children being considered for the study lists serious adverse events associated with the drug, including liver damage, cardiovascular disorders and gastrointestinal problems. However, no mention is made of the increased suicide risk associated with the drug.[34]

None of the other documents provided to parents obtained via FOI informed them of the risk. Curtin University's defence was that it was the responsibility of the paediatricians who diagnosed and prescribed, to inform parents. Curtin invited parents to allow their children to participate and then provided partial information on the risks. They had a responsibility to provide accurate, complete information.

Curtin University defended the conduct of the drug trial. In a statement, Curtin's acting vice-chancellor Linda Kristjanson told the *Australian* newspaper that Curtin's Human Research Ethics Committee was:

> fully informed and was not misled on any aspect of the study. Before approving the study, the university's human research ethics committee conducted a rigorous independent review that complied scrupulously with the National Statement on Ethical Conduct in Research Involving Humans – as prescribed by the National Health and Medical Research Council.[35]

As the acting vice-chancellor indicated, the Human Research Ethics Committee may have been independently aware of the risk of Strattera causing suicidality; the principal researcher, however, the person responsible for the children's drug trial on a day-to-day basis, was ignorant of the significant risks of both the drugs involved in the trial.

In 2006, after Strattera was given its black box warning, one of Curtin's original partners in the study, Sydney's Children's Hospital Education Research Institute advised Associate Professor Jenkins that it was withdrawing as a partner because the Children's Hospital's ethics committee had 'too many objections to put in writing'.[36] Why this did not ring alarm bells at Curtin is an unanswered question. Had it not been for my hearing of Associate Professor Jenkins's evidence to the parliamentary inquiry, and the information uncovered by the Freedom of Information process, these issues would never have seen the light of day. Eli Lilly would have had access to another Strattera study, in this case funded to the tune of $500,000 by Australian taxpayers, supposedly conducted by an independent researcher at a reputable university. How many other supposedly independent studies have been conducted in this way?

Strattera on the PBS

In December 2006 the Commonwealth government's Pharmaceutical Board Advisory Committee (PBAC) advised Eli Lilly that Strattera had been recommended for inclusion on the PBS.[37] Within three weeks of the PBAC recommendation I wrote to Howard government health minister Tony Abbot outlining the history of Strattera and imploring the government not to subsidise Strattera.

The Honourable Christopher Pyne, as the minister assisting Tony Abbott, wrote back defending the PBAC recommendation. He did not address Strattera's record of adverse events or its suicide risk. Instead, he stated that PBAC was an 'independent, expert advisory body' and 'Strattera met all the PBAC criteria for a positive recommendation'. Normally the final decision to approve a drug for inclusion on the PBS is a ministerial decision; however, because of the enormous cost involved

($101.2 million over four years), approval of the full cabinet was required. Approval was granted in April and Strattera was placed on the PBS on 1 July 2007.

Eli Lilly had applied unsuccessfully on at least three previous occasions to have Strattera subsidised via the PBS. In November 2008 I requested, via Freedom of Information, copies of all documents relating to the decision of the PBAC to recommend Strattera's listing on the PBS. I was particularly interested in what consideration had been given by the PBAC to Strattera's black box warning for suicidal ideation and the numerous adverse event reports. The Department of Health and Ageing refused to release all but a tiny percentage of heavily censored and irrelevant documents.

The Administrative Appeals Tribunal heard my appeal in April 2010. The Department of Health and Ageing argued successfully that they had erred in giving me any documents because the *Health Act 1953* prevented anyone working for the Commonwealth revealing information relating to the affairs of a (legal) person (in this case Eli Lilly). The net effect is that the public has no legal right to know why the PBAC recommends taxpayers subsidising any drug. Eli Lilly was the only winner. It benefited from $101.2 million of public funds but the public is not allowed to know why.

The election of the Rudd government in November 2007 led to a false hope that the decision might be reversed and the $101.2 million redirected to interventions that would help and not harm children. I wrote to Nicola Roxon in June 2008 highlighting Strattera's trail of misery and requesting it be removed from the PBS. In response I received a fob-off letter from Minister Roxon's parliamentary secretary, Jan McLucas, defending the process by which the decision to subsidise Strattera was made. The Rudd government had effectively accepted responsibility for the Howard government's poor decision.

How much misery and suffering will children have to endure before Strattera is taken off the Pharmaceutical Benefits Scheme and preferably the market totally? Unlike the ADHD stimulants, Strattera has only been on the market for a few years. It took over seventy years for data about the long-term safety and efficacy of stimulants to become available and even then, it was only by coincidence through the Raine Study data.

If the history of the stimulants is any guide, we can expect to receive the first meaningful data in relation to the long-term safety and efficacy of Strattera in about 2080. Meanwhile, the absence of long-term data should not preclude judgments about whether the known risks of Strattera justify the claimed benefits. The known risks including suicidality and liver failure, as demonstrated by actual incidents of nine-year-old boys attempting suicide and twelve-year-old girls ripping their fingernails and toenails out, surely swamp any temporary improvements in attentiveness and impulsivity.

Appendix 2

Sydney Repeats Perth's Mistakes

Judges are often exposed to the pointy end of prescription amphetamine abuse. In April 2007 New South Wales District Court Judge Paul Conlon, when sentencing a twenty-year-old man said that in his experience ADHD medications were causing significant criminality and drug abuse. 'I have huge concerns. The tide of cases is amazing...I am starting to lose count of [the number of] offenders coming before the courts who were diagnosed at a very young age with ADHD for which they were "medicated".'[1] Judge Conlon also said he had seen signs that children prescribed psychostimulant drugs like Ritalin went on to develop addiction to drugs like methamphetamine. He also expressed frustration at the failure of the medical profession to effectively self regulate:

My own research indicates that ADHD is perhaps the most over-diagnosed condition in today's society...I think it's an absolute disgrace and those doctors and psychiatrists really need to look much more closely at the child and consider other methods of treatment other than putting them on these drugs and chemicals...In other words, they need to apply greater professional rigour.[2]

Then New South Wales health minister Reba Meagher responded to Judge Paul Conlon's comments by setting up a committee to review NSW ADHD diagnosing and prescribing. The review was conducted without public input, and was restricted to a literature review, a survey of prescribers outlining their prescribing practices and a review of the data from the New South Wales Stimulants Committee. The review chairperson Professor Philip Mitchell and two other committee members, Drs Patrick Concannon and Paul Hutchins, have served as advisers to manufacturers of ADHD drugs.[3] In addition, many of the members of the review committee were prescribers who were in effect reviewing their own practice. All of the participants declared their connections to drug manufacturers, but astonishingly claimed there were no conflicts of interest.[4]

Predictably the review concluded that, 'the overall impression was of conscientious doctors giving plenty of time trying to offer the best total management in these very complex situations'.[5] The review, however, was hardly thorough or comprehensive. The audit of patients was restricted to 137 of the 19,382 patients (0.7 per cent) and was a file review only. In other words only the clinician's file notes were reviewed. There was no fresh diagnosis of the children by interviewing parents and teachers. Participation in the audit and the practice survey by prescribers was voluntary, with only 207 of 367 prescribers co-operating.[6] The review described the 56 per cent response rate of prescribers as 'excellent', despite the obvious bias that those who were confident in the rigour of their practices were more likely to participate.[7]

In a disturbing display of ignorance, the review quoted the fourteen-month results of the MTA study as supporting the use of medication while completely disregarding the three-year follow-up results that showed no long-term benefits.[8] (See chapter 2.)

The most worrying aspect of the review, however, was the willingness of clinicians to prescribe a cocktail of psychotropic drugs in conjunction with stimulants. The proportion of other drugs prescribed by surveyed clinicians with stimulants was: Clonidine (75 per cent), atypical antipsychotics (71 per cent), SSRI antidepressants (66 per cent), anti-epileptic medications (55 per cent), tricyclic antidepressants (27 per cent), other anti-depressants (14 per cent) and conventional antipsychotics (12 per cent).[9] Some of these drugs are contraindicated for use with stimulants and/or are not recommended for use in children.

The prescribing patterns were similar to those in Western Australia, with a minority of prescribers specialising in ADHD.[10] The review also confirmed that New South Wales paediatricians, like their Western Australian colleagues, were far more likely to be frequent prescribers than a child psychiatrist.[11] The review report stated that:

> many of the children and families were battling with
> very complex situations…many children had signifi-
> cant learning difficulties, social problems, and other

developmental conditions and were living in dysfunctional and sometimes chaotic families, including
changes in carers. Several children were being reared
by grandparents and a number were in foster homes or
experiencing multiple placements. Domestic violence
and parental substance abuse were not uncommon.[12]

Typical of ADHD industry approach, these complexities were
in practice ignored with pharmaceutical interventions being the
simple solution to life's complexities.

Given Professor Mitchell's and Drs Hutchins's and
Concannon's pharmaceutical company connections, the findings of the review were hardly suprising. The treatment of Judge
Conlon following his comments, however, was alarming and
reflects the desperation to shut down debate. On 25 February
2008, the *Daily Telegraph* reported that as a result of a complaint
by an undisclosed ADHD support group, Judge Conlon was
'gagged' from making further comments on his experience of
ADHD medications leading to drug abuse and criminality.[13]
Judge Conlon had called on the medical profession to apply
greater 'professional vigour'. His reward was a 'gag' and a white-
wash review by ADHD proponents.

During the 1990s and through to 2003, Western Australian
child prescribing rates were much higher than New South
Wales rates.[14] Since 2003 Western Australian rates have fallen
dramatically while rates in New South Wales have skyrocketed.
In 2007 child prescribing rates were roughly equivalent.[15] Since
2007 New South Wales total PBS-subsidised prescription rates
have more than doubled.[16] While there are no actual figures for
WA or NSW later than 2007, all the available evidence strongly

indicates per capita child prescribing rates in NSW now exceed those in WA. Everything that is happening in Sydney has happened and been exposed in Perth. Sydney hasn't learned from Perth's mistakes; it is repeating them.

Notes

Introduction: Martin's ADHD Journey

1   Name changed to protect anonymity.

Chapter 1: Diagnosis: Disease, Disorder or Difference?

1   Lisa Cosgrove, Sheldon Krimsky and Manisha Vijayaraghavan,
     'Financial Ties between DSM-IV Panel Members and the
     Pharmaceutical Industry', *Psychotherapy and Psychosomatics,* 75, 2006,
     p. 154; American Psychiatric Association, *Diagnostic and Statistical
     Manual of Mental Disorders,* Fourth Edition, Text Revision, American
     Psychiatric Association, Washington DC, 2000.

2   American Psychiatric Association, *Diagnostic and Statistical Manual
     of Mental Disorders,* pp. 88–89.

3   ibid.

4   ibid., p. 85.

5   ibid., pp. 92–93.

6   ibid., pp. 86–87.

7   Some of the most common conditions diagnosed with ADHD are:
     depression, bipolar disorder, anxiety disorder, learning disabilities,
     conduct disorder, oppositional defiant disorder, sleep disorders,
     Tourette disorder, pervasive developmental disorder and obsessive
     compulsive disorder.

Carol E. Watkins, MD, *AD/HD and Comorbidity: What's Under the Tip of the Iceberg*?, http://www.baltimorepsych.com/ADD_Comorbidity. htm (accessed on 1 March 2007).

8   Michelle Wiese Bockmann, 'General Ritalin', *The Australian,* 19 September 2005.

9   Sarah Ferguson and Nick Rushworth, 'ADHD – The Quick Fix', *The Sunday Program*, Channel 9, 14 May 2006. Interview previously available at http://sunday.ninemsn.com.au/sunday/cover_stories/article_1983.asp?s=1 (accessed 2 April 2008).

10 Colleen Egan, 'Drugging Our Young', *The Sunday Times,* 11 July 2004.

11 Fred A. Baughman Jr., MD and Craig Hovey, *The ADHD Fraud: How Psychiatry Makes 'Patients' of Normal Children*, Trafford Publishing, Victoria BC, 2006, pp. 52–53.

12 ibid. p. 54.

13 In 1991 in Australia, less than 10,000 prescriptions were dispensed for dexamphetamine sulphate. In 1998, nearly 250,000 prescriptions were dispensed for the same drug, an increase of 2400 per cent. Paul Mackey and Andrew Kopras, *Medication for Attention Deficit Hyperactivity Disorder (ADHD): An Analysis by Federal Electorate,* Parliament of Australia, Canberra, 2001, p. 4.

14 Baughman Jr., and Hovey, *The ADHD Fraud*, p. 58.

15 Dr Allen Frances, 'Psychiatrists Propose Revisions to Diagnosis Manual', *PBS Newshour*, 10 February 2010. Available at http://www.pbs.org/newshour/bb/health/jan-june10/mentalillness_02-10.html (accessed 26 February 2010).

16 Dawn Gibson, 'Quiet children slip ADHD net', *The West Australian,* 16 April 2003.

17 Michelle Toner, *Fact Sheet: ADHD in Adults,* Learning and Attentional Disorders Society of WA Inc, Perth, 2003.

18 Department of Health, Government of Western Australia, *Inquiry into Attention Deficit Disorder and Attention Deficit Hyperactivity Disorder in Western Australia,* Legislative Assembly, Transcript of evidence taken on 27 October 2003, p. 2 (Michelle Toner).

19 Russell A. Barkley, et al., 'International Consensus Statement on ADHD', *Clinical Child and Family Psychology Review*, Vol 5, No. 2, June 2002, p. 89.

20 Sami Timimi, et al., 'A Critique of the International Consensus Statement on ADHD', *Clinical Child and Family Psychology Review,* Vol. 7, No. 1, 2004, p. 59.

21 ibid.

22 ibid., p. 60.

23 Peter R. Breggin, M.D., *Talking Back to Ritalin: What Doctors Aren't Telling You about Stimulants for Children,* Common Courage Press, Monroe, 1998, p. 358.

24 'Despite significant advances in the state of the art, the potential clinical applications of neuroimaging research to the psychiatric care of children has yet to be realized.' Gahan J. Pandina, 'Review of Neuroimaging Studies of Child Adolescent Psychiatric Disorders from the past 10 years (Statistical Data Included)', *Journal of the American Academy of Child & Adolescent Psychiatry,* Vol. 39 No. 7, July 2000, pp. 815–28.

25 'Although gross differences in size or symmetry of brain structures can be quantified, individual cells and cell layers cannot yet be visualized. This means that, although the volume and shape of brain structures may be determined, the underlying cause of any differences cannot.' Sarah Durston, Hilleke E. Hulshoff Pol, B. J. Casey, Jay N. Giedd, Jan K. Buitelaar, Herman van Engeland, 'Anatomical MRI of the Developing Human Brain: What Have We Learned?', *Journal of the American Academy of Child & Adolescent Psychiatry,* Vol. 40 Issue 9, September 2001, pp. 1012–20.

26 Bob Jacobs, Youth Affairs Network of Queensland, *Being an Educated Consumer of 'ADHD' Research,* Youth Affairs Network of Queensland, 2005.

27 Larry S. Goldman, Myron Genel, Rebecca J. Bezman, Priscilla J. Slanetz, for the Council on Scientific Affairs, American Medical Association, 'Diagnosis and treatment of attention-deficit/hyperactivity disorder in children and adolescents', *Journal of the American Medical Association,* 279(14), pp. 1100–07.

28 Professor Stephen Houghton, Psychologist/University Professor, Graduate School of Education, University of Western Australia, transcript of evidence given to Inquiry into Attention Deficit Disorder and Attention Deficit Hyperactivity Disorder in Western Australia, in Perth on 26 November 2003.

29 M. G. Sawyer, F. M. Arney, et al., *The Mental Health of Young People in Australia,* Mental Health and Special Programs Branch, Commonwealth Department of Health and Aged Care, Canberra 2000, p. 809.

30 'The mental disorders were assessed using the parent-version of the Diagnostic Interview Schedule for Children Version IV. Parents completed the Child Behaviour Checklist to identify mental health problems and standard questionnaires to assess health-related quality

of life and service use. The Youth Risk Behaviour Questionnaire completed by adolescents was employed to identify health-risk behaviours.' M. G. Sawyer, R. J. Kosky et al., 'The National Survey of Mental Health and Wellbeing: the child and adolescent component' in *Australian and New Zealand Journal of Psychiatry*, 34, 2000, p. 215.

31 Salynn Boyles, 'Study confirms ADHD is more common in boys', *WebMD Health News*, 15 September 2004. Available at http://www.webmd.com/add-adhd/news/20040915/study-confirms-adhd-is-more-common-in-boys (accessed 4 October 2009).

32 Belinda Hickman, 'AMA backs drug complaints', *The Australian*, 20 December 2002.

33 The Hon. Nicola Roxon MP, National Health and Medical Research Council, and Royal Australasian College of Physicians, *Draft ADHD Guidelines Released*, Joint Media Release, 30 November 2009.

Chapter 2: Amphetamine Deficit Disorder

1 David Keirsey, 'The Great A.D.D. Hoax' at Keirsey.com, n.d., http://www.keirsey.com/add_hoax.aspx (accessed 20 March 2008).

2 Other less commonly used brand names for methylphenidate include Methylin, Daytrana, Rubifen, Equasym and Metadate.

3 Lydia Furman, 'What is Attention-Deficit Hyperactivity Disorder (ADHD)?', *Journal of Child Neurology*, Vol. 20 No. 12, 2005, p. 998.

4 Breggin, *Talking Back to Ritalin*, p. 20.

5 J. L. Rapoport, M. S. Buchsbaum, et al., 'Dextroamphetamine: cognitive and behavioural effects in normal prepubertal boys', *Science*, Vol. 199, No. 4323, (3 February 1978), p. 561. The dose was 0.5mg/kg.

6 Breggin, *Talking Back to Ritalin*, p. 22.

7 Baughman Jr. and Hovey, *The ADHD Fraud*, p. 6.

8 Furman, 'What is Attention-Deficit Hyperactivity Disorder (ADHD)?'

9 Egan, 'Drugging Our Young'.

10 'Always on the Go' in *Openmind 123*, October/September 2003. Available at http://www.bonkers.hall.btinternet.co.uk/openmind.html (accessed 24 August 2006).

11 Russell A. Barkley was the first signatory to the International Consensus Statement on ADHD. See Barkley, et al., 'International Consensus Statement on ADHD', p. 91.

12 Quoted in Baughman Jr., and Hovey, *The ADHD Fraud*, p. 33.

13 Barkley and Cunningham (1979). Quoted in Breggin, *Talking Back to Ritalin*, p. 59.

14   Breggin, *Talking Back to Ritalin*, pp. 58–60.

15   ibid., p. 186.

16   American Psychiatric Association, *Treatments of Psychiatric Disorders: a task force report of the American Psychiatric Association,* 1st ed., 1989, quoted in ibid., p. 71.

17   American Psychiatric Association, *Diagnostic and Statistical Manual of Mental Disorders,* Fourth Edition, Text Revision, American Psychiatric Association, Washington DC, 2000, p. 223.

18   ibid., p. 225.

19   GlaxoSmithKline, *Prescribing Information – Dexedrine (dextroamphetamine sulphate).* Available at http://www.gskus.com/products/assets/ us_dexedrine.pdf (accessed 28 July 2009).

20   Parliament of Western Australia, *Hansard,* Martin Whitely MLA, Thursday, 25 February 2010, pp. 259b–293a.

21   For instance, see Dave Coghill, 'Attention-deficit hyperactivity disorder: should we believe the mass media or peer-reviewed literature?', *The Psychiatrist,* 29, 2005, pp. 288–91; Dr Ken Whiting, *Fact Sheet: Attention Deficit/Hyperactivity Disorder 2003 Update,* Learning and Attentional Disorders Society of WA, Perth, 2003.

22   From 1995-2004 Western Australia had the highest rate of illicit drug abuse of any Australian state. The rates of abuse of amphetamines were also the highest in Australia. Source: 2004 National Drug Strategy Household survey, State and Territory Supplement. Australian Institute of Health and Welfare, Canberra, 2005.

23   1999 Australian School Students Alcohol and Drugs Survey quoted in Kate Gauntlett, 'Drugs so easy to find', *The West Australian,* 14 June 2003.

24   The 2008 Australian Secondary Students' Alcohol and Drug Survey (ASSAD) data indicated a reduction in 'last 12 month amphetamine abuse' by school children 12–17 years old from 10.3 per cent in 2002, 6.5 per cent in 2005, and 5.1 per cent in 2008. P. Griffiths, R. Kalic, & A. Gunnell, *Australian School Student Survey 2008: Western Australian Results (excluding tobacco),* Brief Communication no. 2, Drug and Alcohol Office, Perth, 2009.

25   Drug and Alcohol Office WA, *ASSAD Drug Report 2005,* Mt Lawley, March 2007, pp. 30–32.

26   ibid. p. 33.

27   ibid.

28   Clare Trevelyan, 'Coming Down', *The West Australian,* 27 February 2010.

29 Western Australia, *Parliamentary Debates,* Legislative Assembly, 2 June 2005, p. 2687b–2708a (Martin Whitely, Member for Bassendean).

30 Western Australia, *Parliamentary Debates,* Legislative Assembly, 27 September 2007, p. 5946 (Alan Carpenter, Premier).

31 Breggin, *Talking Back to Ritalin,* p. 69.

32 Federal Drug Administration, *Statement on Concerta and Methylphenidate for the June 30 PAC,* Available at http://www.fda.gov/ohrms/ dockets/ac/05/briefing/2005-4152b1_00_05a_Statement%20for%20 June%2030.pdf (accessed 11 April 2008).

33 Drug and Alcohol Office, *Dexamphetamine: Facts,* Prevention Branch, Drug and Alcohol Office, Perth, 2002, p. 3.

34 Commonwealth Department of Health and Aged Care, Australian Bureau of Statistics, *Population by Age and Sex,* June 2000 (ABS 3201.0).

35 Australian Institute of Health and Welfare, *2004 National Drug Strategy Household Survey: State and territory supplement,* AIHW cat. No. PHE 61, Canberra, AIHW, 2005, p. 7.

36 Australian Institute of Health and Welfare, *Alcohol and other drug treatment services in Australia 2005-06,* Drug Treatment Series, Number 7, Australian Institute of Health and Welfare, Canberra, July 2007, p. 14.

37 GlaxoSmithKline, *Prescribing Information – Dexedrine (dextroamphetamine sulphate),* July 2008. Available at http://www.gskus.com/products/ assets/us_dexedrine.pdf (accessed 28 July 2009).

38 Consumer Medicine Information for Ritalin, Concerta and Attenta can be found at the following websites: Ritalin: http://www.pharma.us.novartis.com/product/pi/pdf/ ritalin_ritalin-sr.pdf; Concerta: http://www.concerta.net/assets/Prescribing_Info-short.pdf; Attenta: http://www.nps.org.au/__data/assets/pdf_file/0018/13464/ afcatten.pdf.

39 Adverse events information related to Strattera obtained from the Therapeutic Goods Administration's Public Case Detail reports.

40 Con Berbatis, 'Primary care and Pharmacy: 4. Large contributions to national adverse reaction reporting by pharmacists in Australia', *i2P E-Magazine,* Issue 72, June 2008, p. 1.

41 ADEC's committee is appointed by the Minister for Health and Ageing and provides advice to the Minister and the Secretary of the Commonwealth Department of Health and Ageing through the Therapeutic Goods Administration, on the quality, risk-benefit, and

effectiveness of any drug referred to it for evaluation. Available at http://www.tga.gov.au/docs/html/adec/adec.htm.

42   Australian Drug Evaluation Committee, *Evaluation of Clinical Data, Part IV,* Meeting No. 1993/2, 10 March 1993. Obtained through *Freedom of Information Act 1992.*

43   Australian Government, Written Question on Notice, *Ritalin,* Budget Estimates 2006-2007, 31 May–1 June 2006.

44   Federal Drug Administration, *Statement on Concerta and Methylphenidate for the June 30 PAC.* Available at http://www.fda.gov/ohrms/dockets/ac/05/briefing/2005-4152b1_00_05a_Statement%20for%20June%2030.pdf (accessed 11 April 2008).

45   Lisa Allen, 'Attention deficit drugs in spotlight', *Australian Financial Review,* 1 July 2005.

46   Australian Government, *Therapeutic Goods Amendment (Repeal of Ministerial Responsibility for Approval of RU486) Bill 2005,* Community Affairs Legislation Committee, 3 February 2006.

47   'The TGA does not record which drugs sold in the US, with black box warnings in the US approved prescribing information document, do not carry black box warnings in the Australian prescribing information (P1) document'. Australian Government, Written Question on Notice, *Black Box Warnings,* Budget Estimates 2006–2007, 31 May–1 June 2006.

48   H. Schacter, B. Pham, J. King, S. Langford, & D. Mother, 'How efficacious and safe is short-acting methylphenidate for the treatment of attention–deficit disorder in children and adolescents? A meta-analysis', *Canadian Medical Association Journal,* 165, 2001, pp. 1475–1488. Available at http://www.cmaj.ca/cgi/content/full/165/11/1475 (accessed 10 March 2008).

49   Marian S. McDonagh, Kim Petersen, et al., *Drug Class Review on Pharmacologic Treatments for ADHD: Final Report Update 2,* Portland, Oregon Health & Science University (2007). Available at http://www.ohsu.edu/ohsuedu/research/policycenter/customcf/derp/product/ADHD_Final%20Report%20Update%202_Evidence%20Tables.pdf (accessed 13 February 2009).

50   Alexander Otto, 'Are ADHD drugs safe? Report finds little proof', *The News Tribune,* 13 September 2005. Available at http://www.playattention.com/attention-deficit/articles/are-adhd-drugs-safe-report-finds-little-proof (accessed 12 May 2007).

51   ibid.

52   ibid.

53   Oregon Health & Science University, *Drug Class Review on Pharmacologic Treatments for ADHD,* Portland, Oregon, 2007, p. 24.

54   ibid., p. 20.

55   ibid., p. 16.

56   ibid., p. 19.

57   ibid., p. 21.

58   The senior vice president of the Pharmaceutical Research and Manufacturers of America, Ken Johnson, refused to comment directly on the Oregon Review, but offered the standard ADHD industry response that the use of drugs to treat ADHD clearly outweighed the risks. Cited in Otto, 'Are ADHD drugs safe? Report finds little proof'.

59   Finding 13, Western Australia Legislative Assembly, *Attention Deficit Hyperactivity Disorder in Western Australia,* Education and Health Standing Committee, Report No. 8, 2004, p. 42.

60   As early as the 1930s, low doses of stimulant drugs were used to try to modify the behaviour of children with these diagnoses.' Earl Mindell and Virginia Hopkins, *Alternatives: Hundreds of safe, natural, prescription-free remedies to restore and maintain your health,* McGraw Hill, New York, 2009.

61   Peter Breggin, 'A Critical Analysis of the NIMH Multimodal Treatment Study for Attention-Deficit/Hyperactivity Disorder (The MTA Study)' in *Psychiatric Drug Facts* 2000. Available at http://www.breggin.com/mta.html (accessed March 20 2008); The MTA Study was 'the first multisite, cooperative agreement treatment study of children, and the largest psychiatric/psychological treatment trial ever conducted by the (U.S.) National Institute of Mental Health. It examines the effectiveness of Medication vs. Psychosocial treatment vs. their combination for treatment of ADHD and compares these experimental arms to each other and to routine community care.' K. C. Wells, W. E. Pelham, et al., 'Psychosocial treatment strategies in the MTA study: rationale, methods, and critical issues in design and implementation', (abstract), *Journal of Abnormal Child Psychology,* Vol. 28, No. 6, 2000. Available at http://www.ncbi.nlm.nih.gov/pubmed/11104313 (accessed 7 February 2008).

62   The study was sponsored by the National Institute of Mental Health (NIMH) and conducted at six separate US sites. At each site, the study compared four treatment conditions: medication management alone, combined medication management and behavioural therapy, behavioural therapy, and community care. The average age of the children was eight and 80 per cent were boys. For more information,

see The MTA Cooperative Group, 'A 14-Month Randomized Clinical Trial of Treatment Strategies for Attention-Deficit/ Hyperactivity Disorder', *Archives of General Psychiatry,* 56, 1999, p. 1073.

63 Merle G. Paule, Andrew S. Rowland, Sherry A. Ferguson, et al., 'Attention deficit/hyperactivity disorder: characteristics, interventions, and models' in *Neurotoxicology and Teratology,* Vol. 22, No. 5, 2000, p. 631. Available at http://cat.inist.fr/?aModele=afficheN&cps idt=1030283 (accessed 13 February 2009).

64 Allegra Stratton, 'Questions raised about drugs as treatment for ADHD sufferers', *The Guardian,* November 12th, 2007. Available at http://www.thefooddoctor.com (accessed 26 March 2008).

65 Brooke Molina, Kate Flory, Stephen P. Hinshaw et al., 'Delinquent Behavior and Emerging Substance Use in the MTA at 36 Months: Prevalence, Course, and Treatment Effects', *Journal of the American Academy of Child & Adolescent Psychiatry,* Vol. 46 No. 8, August 2007: pp. 1028–1040; Stratton, 'Questions raised about drugs as treatment for ADHD sufferers'.

66 Joseph M. Rey, 'In the long run, skills are as good as pills for attention deficit hyperactivity disorder', *The Medical Journal of Australia,* 188:3, 2008, p. 134.

67 The Raine Study started in 1989, when 2900 pregnant women were recruited into a comprehensive health and wellbeing research study at King Edward Memorial Hospital to examine ultrasound imaging. The mothers were assessed during pregnancy and after the children were born, and at one year, then two, three and five years of age. Information on their height, weight, eating, walking, talking, eating, behaviour, any medical conditions or illness etc. was collected. Further follow ups of the cohort have been conducted at eight, ten, fourteen, and seventeen years of age. At each follow-up information is collected from the parents and the child. The current follow up is being done at twenty years of age. By age fourteen 'of the 1785 adolescents (remaining) in the sample, 131 (7.3 per cent) had received a diagnosis of ADHD'. At age five none of the 131 had taken ADHD stimulants. By age fourteen, twenty-nine had never taken stimulants, forty-one had been on prescription stimulants in the past but were not taking them, and sixty-one were on ADHD stimulants. This gave three groups for comparison, the 'never medicated', 'previously medicated' and the 'currently medicated' groups. In addition analysis of the effect of the duration of stimulant treatment was undertaken. Available at http://www.rainestudy.org.au (accessed 7 May 2010).

The statistically significant differences that existed at age fourteen occurred between age five and fourteen, after some of the children were medicated. To the extent that (non-statistically significant differences) existed at age five these were 'controlled for by using the "propensity for medication" score, the symptom severity before commencement of medication treatment, and a number of sociodemographic measures'.

68 Government of Western Australia, Department of Health, *Raine ADHD Study: Long-term outcomes associated with stimulant medication in the treatment of ADHD in children,* Department of Health, Perth, 2010.

69 ibid., p. 52.

70 ibid., p. 6.

71 ibid., p. 5

72 ibid., p. 30; The short term studies referred to in the Raine Study are Howard B. Abikoff, et al., 'Methylphenidate effects on Functional Outcomes in the Preschoolers with Attention-Deficit/Hyperactivity Disorder Treatment Study (PATS)', *Journal of Child and Adolescent Psychopharmacology,* 17(5), 2007, pp. 581–92; C. L. Carlson & M. R. Bunner, 'Effects of Methylphenidate on the Academic Performance of Children with Attention-Deficit Hyperactivity Disorder and Learning Disabilities', *School Psychology Review,* 22(2), 1993, pp. 184–98; Irene M. Loe & Heidi M. Feldman, 'Academic and educational outcomes of children with ADHD', *Journal of Pediatric Psychology,* 32(6), 2007, pp. 643–54.

73 Interview with Professor Ian Hickie on ABC *PM* program with Mark Colvin, 'New Research Reignites Debate over ADHD', 17 February 2002. Available at http://www.abc.net.au/pm/content/2010/s2822748. htm (accessed 15 March 2010).

74 Professor Ian Hickie received the following grants totalling $411,000 from pharmaceutical companies: $10,000 from Roche Pharmaceuticals (1992); $30,000 from Bristol-Myers Squibb (1997); $40,000 from Bristol-Myers Squibb (1998–1999); $250,000 from Pfizer Australia (2009); $81,000 from Pfizer Australia (n.d.). Cited in Ian Hickie, Curriculum Vitae, last updated 23 August 2009.

75 Government of Western Australia, Department of Health, *Study raises questions about long-term effect of ADHD* medication, Media Release, 17 February 2010.

Chapter 3: True Believers

1 Leonard Sax, 'Ritalin: Better Living Through Chemistry?', *The World and I Online,* November 2000, pp. 287-99, http://www.worldandi.

com/public/2000/november/sax.html (accessed 2 April 2008).

2 Breggin, *Talking Back to Ritalin,* p. 188.

3 Egan, 'Drugging Our Young'.

4 Cathy O'Leary, 'Violent tots need taming before it's too late: expert', *The West Australian,* 3 February 2006.

5 ibid.

6 Kenneth Whiting, 'Attention Deficit/Hyperactivity Disorder', *The Australian Crime Prevention Council, 20th Biennial Conference on Preventing Crime,* Fremantle, 21–22 March 1995.

7 Egan, 'Drugging Our Young'.

8 Ferguson and Rushworth, 'ADHD – The Quick Fix'.

9 Western Australia Legislative Assembly, *Attention Deficit Hyperactivity Disorder in Western Australia,* Education and Health Standing Committee, Report No. 8, 2004, p. 45.

10 Ferguson and Rushworth, 'ADHD – The Quick Fix'.

11 In 2004 a survey revealed that 'two-thirds of global health charities and patient groups now accept support from drug or device manufacturers.' Quoted in Ray Moynihan and Alan Cassels, *Selling Sickness: How the World's Biggest Pharmaceutical Companies Are Turning us all into Patients,* Nation Books, New York, 2005, p. 62.

12 Moynihan and Cassels, *Selling Sickness,* pp. 66–67.

13 ibid., p. 67.

14 Kelly Patricia O'Meara, 'Putting Power Back in Parental Hands; legislation being considered that would allow parents not schools to decide whether their children need to be medicated as a prerequisite for attending classes', *Washington Post's Insight Magazine,* 26 May 2003.

15 Breggin, *Talking Back to Ritalin,* p. 236.

16 Paul H. Wender, *Attention-Deficit Hyperactivity Disorder in Adults,* Oxford University Press, New York, 1995, p. 20.

17 ibid., pp. 139–49.

18 'LADS has accepted limited unrestricted grants from pharmaceutical companies.' (Including Eli Lilly and Novartis.) See http://www.ladswa.com.au/page.php?id=6 (accessed 26 June 2009).

19 Derek Cohen (ed.), *Fact Sheet: Parenting a Child with ADHD,* Learning and Attentional Disorders Society of WA Inc, Perth, n.d.

20 'Help for ADHD sufferers', *Medical & Healthy Living, Community Newspaper,* Perth, 20 September 2004.

21 Dr Roger Patterson interviewed on *Face the Facts,* video recording taken from Channel 31 Perth, 27 January 2003.

22 Michelle Toner interviewed on, *Face the Facts,* video recording taken from Channel 31 Perth, 27 January 2003. This information is also

referred to in Ferguson and Rushworth, 'ADHD – The Quick Fix'.

23 'Individual patient response to amphetamines varies widely. While toxic symptoms occasionally occur as an idiosyncrasy at doses as low as 2mg, they are rare with doses of less than 15mg; 30mg can produce severe reactions, yet doses of 400 to 500mg are not necessarily fatal.' GlaxoSmithKline's Prescribing Information for Dexedrine (dextroamphetamine sulphate). Available at http://us.gsk.com/products/assets/us_dexedrine.pdf (accessed 26 June 2009).

24 Toner interview, *Face the Facts*.

25 Beata Silber, Katherine Papafotiou et al., 'The effects of dexamphetamine on simulated driving performance', *Psychopharmacology*, 179, 2005, pp. 541–42.

26 WA Stimulant Committee, Minutes of Meeting held on 4 August, 1998, obtained under *Freedom of Information Act 1992*.

27 Last Say Communications, *ADHD – A Day of Calm – Dawn to Dusk: Long Lasting Medication to Provide Relief for Kids with ADHD*, Media Release, 27 March 2007.

28 Linda Graham, 'The Politics of ADHD', in *Proceedings of the Australian Association for Research in Education (AARE) Annual Conference*, Adelaide, November 2006, p. 14.

29 American Psychiatric Association, *Diagnostic and Statistical Manual of Mental Disorders*, Fourth Edition, p. 87.

30 Egan, 'Drugging Our Young'.

31 Verbal interview conducted by author with Paul Andrews MLA, Member for Southern River, Parliament of Western Australia, 26 February 2008.

32 Linda J. Graham, 'Drugs, labels and (p)ill-fitting boxes: ADHD and children who are hard to teach', in *Discourse: Studies in the Cultural Politics of Education*, Vol. 29, No. 1, March 2008, p. 94.

33 Ronald Lipman, 'Federal involvement in the use of behaviour modification drugs on grammar school children of the right to privacy inquiry. Hearing before a Subcommittee of the Committee on Government Operations House of Representatives, Ninety-First Congress, Second Session, 29 September 1970, p. 33. Available at http://www.fredsworld02.com/pdf/federal%20involvement.pdf (accessed 9 April 2008).

34 Graham, 'Drugs, labels and (p)ill-fitting boxes'.

35 Daryl Passmore, 'Out of Control', *Courier Mail*, 14 January 2007. Available at http://www.news.com.au/couriermail/story/0,,21052984-23272,00.html (accessed 24 June 2009).

36 Graham, 'Drugs, labels and (p)ill-fitting boxes', p. 95.

37   ibid.

38   Fifty-six per cent of the GPs polled thought that ADHD drugs were
     over-prescribed to children in Western Australia and some 16 per
     cent thought they were not. The other 28 per cent of GPs basically
     did not express an opinion. Rob McEvoy, 'Poll Results – General
     Practitioners May 2006', *Medical.WA Forum,* 2 May 2006. Available
     at http://www.medicalhub.com.au/index.php?option=com_
     docman&task=doc_download&gid=84 (accessed 17 June 2007).

39   Some notable exceptions include Drs Jon Juredeini and Gil Anaf (SA),
     Dr George Halasz (Vic) and Drs Lois Achimovich, Joe Kosterich, Lou
     Landau, Helen Milroy, Kathy Nottage and the late Dr Mark Rooney
     (WA). Apologies to others not mentioned who advocated to end or
     reduce the reliance on ADHD medications for managing childhood
     behaviours.

Chapter 4: Uncle Sam Knows Best

1   'The use of different diagnostic tools may explain the variation in
     ADHD prevalence rates between Australia (DSM-IV) and the United
     Kingdom (ICD-10).' Western Australia Legislative Assembly, *Attention
     Deficit Hyperactivity Disorder in Western Australia,* Education and Health
     Standing Committee, Report No. 8, 2004, p. 14; Constantine
     G. Berbatis, V. Bruce Sunderland et al., 'Licit psychostimulant
     consumption in Australia, 1984–2000: international and jurisdictional
     comparison', *Medical Journal of Australia,* 177; 10, 2002, p. 540; 'The
     DSM-IV allows for multiple diagnosis with co-morbid conditions such
     as conduct disorder, while ICD-10 does not…As a result, prevalence
     studies from other countries using the ICD-10 (e.g. UK) indicate
     much lower ADHD rates than those from Australia and the USA.'
     Parliament of South Australia, *Inquiry into Attention Deficit Hyperactivity
     Disorder: Sixteenth Report of the Social Development Committee,* Legislative
     Council, 2002, p. 12.

2   Merete Juul Sorenson, Ole Mors and Per Hove Thomsen, 'DSM-IV
     or ICD-10-DCR diagnoses in child and adolescent psychiatry: does it
     matter?, *European Journal of Child and Adolescent Psychiatry,* 14; 6 (Sept
     2005): p. 339.

3   ibid.

4   The criteria for this disorder state that 'Mathematics disorder, formerly
     called developmental arithmetic disorder, developmental acalculia, or
     dyscalculia, is a learning disorder in which a person's mathematical
     ability is substantially below the level normally expected based on his
     or her age, intelligence, life experiences, educational background, and

physical impairments.' American Psychiatric Association, *Diagnostic and Statistical Manual of Mental Disorders*, Fourth Edition, p. 53.

5　Breggin, *Talking Back to Ritalin*, p. 216.

6　Quoted in ibid., p. 215.

7　Joseph Glenmullen, *Prozac Backlash: Overcoming the Dangers of Prozac, Zoloft, Paxil, and other Antidepressants with Safe, Effective Alternatives*, Simon & Schuster, New York, 2000, p. 196.

8　'Respondents Urge Caution When Using the DSM-IV,' *Clinical Psychiatry News*, 28(1): 14, 2000.

9　'For several years, Grassley has conducted extensive oversight and sought disclosure of financial ties with industry from research physicians, medical schools, medical journals, continuing medical education, and the patient advocacy community. He has worked to expose cases where there was vast disparity between drug-company payments received and reported by leading medical researchers. In response to Grassley's work, the National Institute of Health is working on new disclosure guidelines for federal grant recipients. Grassley is also working for congressional passage of reform legislation he has sponsored with Senator Herb Kohl. Their bipartisan Physician Payments Sunshine Act would require annual public reporting by drug, device and biologic manufacturers of payments made to physicians nationwide.' Senator Chuck Grassley of Iowa, 'Grassley works for disclosure of drug company payments to medical groups', 8 December 2009. Available at http://grassley.senate.gov/news/Article. cfm?customel_dataPageID_1502=24413# (accessed 28 March 2010).

10　Gardiner Harris and Benedict Carey, 'Psychiatric Group Faces Scrutiny Over Drug Industry Ties,' *The New York Times*, 12 July 2008.

11　Dan Vergano, 'Medical manual's authors often tied to drugmakers', *USA Today*, 19 April, 2008. Available at http://www.usatoday.com/ news/health/2006-04-19-manuals-drugmakers_x.htm (accessed 21 June 2009).

12　Harris and Carey, 'Psychiatric Group Faces Scrutiny Over Drug Industry Ties'.

13　Steven S. Sharfstein, 'Big Pharma and American Psychiatry', *Psychiatric News*, Vol. 40, No. 16, August 2008, p. 3.

14　Dr Allen Frances, 'Psychiatrists Propose Revisions to Diagnosis Manual', *PBS Newshour*, 10 February 2010. Available at http://www. pbs.org/newshour/bb/health/jan-june10/mentalillness_02-10.html (accessed 26 February 2010).

15 Breggin, *Talking Back to Ritalin*, p. 286.
16 David Armstrong and Keith J. Winstein, 'Antidepressants Under Scrutiny Over Efficacy', *The Wall Street Journal*, 17 January 2008.
17 ibid.
18 ibid.
19 Breggin, *Talking Back to Ritalin*, p. 264.
20 ibid., p. 265.
21 ibid.
22 ibid., p. 266.
23 Gardiner Harris, 'Regulation Redefined: At F.D.A., Strong Drug Ties and Less Monitoring', *The New York Times*, 6 December 2004. Available at http://www.nytimes.com/2004/12/06/health/06fda. html?_r=1&pagewanted=print&position= (accessed 25 October 2008).
24 ibid.
25 Breggin, *Talking Back to Ritalin*, p. 186.
26 A black box warning is a recognition of how harmful the drug can be if given to patients who are at risk of developing the possible adverse side effects. The name derives from the warning being surrounded by a printed black box. See Trisha Torrey, 'Black Box Warning (From the FDA)', August 2008. Available at http://patients.about.com/od/ glossary/g/blackboxwarning.htm (accessed 18 March 2010).
27 Gardiner Harris, 'Warning Urged on Stimulants Like Ritalin', *The New York Times*, 10 February 2006. Available at http://www. nytimes.com/2006/02/10/health/policy/10drug.html?ei=5090& en=88c174fed7f7f6ff&ex=1297227600&partner=rssuserland&em c=rss&pagewanted=print (accessed 26 October 2008); Associated Press, 'Feds Recommend Warnings on ADHD Drugs', Fox News. com, 10 February 2006. Available at http://www.foxnews.com/ story/0,2933,184447,00.html?sPage=fnc/us/lawcenter (accessed 27 September 2006).
28 Medwire News, 'Warning proposed for ADHD drugs', *MedWire News, General Medicine*, 10 February 2006. Available at http://www. medwire-news.md/news/article.aspx?k=51&id=54145 (accessed 25 October 2009).
29 Gardiner Harris, 'F.D.A. Panel Urges Warnings on Ritalin and Other Stimulants' *The New York Times*, 9 February 2006. Available at http:// www.nytimes.com/2006/02/10/health/policy/10drug.html?ei=5090 &en=88c174fed7f7f6ff&ex=1297227600&partner=rssuserland&emc=r ss&pagewanted=print (accessed 26 October 2008).
30 Vioxx was an arthritis and acute pain medication that was launched in

the United States in 1999 by Merck & Co and was marketed in over eighty countries. Sales in 2003 were worth $2.5 billion. In March 2000 the results of a study, the Vioxx Gastrointestinal Outcomes Research (VIGOR), indicated an increased risk of cardiovascular events. This trial found that there was an increased relative risk for confirmed cardiovascular events, such as heart attack and stroke, 18 months after treatment began. 'Merck Announces Voluntary Worldwide Withdrawal of VIOXX®', available at http://www.merck.com/newsroom/vioxx/pdf/vioxx_press_release_final.pdf (accessed 7 February 2007). Merck failed to warn treating doctors or patients about the results of the VIGOR study (2000). No information, let alone warnings, about the risks were given, until some two years later. Even then the information that was finally given was unclear. Consequently, doctors and patients continued prescribing and using Vioxx until its withdrawal. As a result, thousands of people may have suffered serious injury.

31 Amanda Gardner, 'FDA Panel Calls for Strongest Warning on ADHD drugs', *Healthday News,* 9 February 2006.

32 ibid.

33 Harris, 'Warning Urged on Stimulants Like Ritalin'.

34 ibid.

35 Andrew Bridges, 'Advisers Reject Strong ADHD Warnings', *ABC News*, Washington DC, 2006, quoted in Graham, 'Drugs, labels and (p)ill-fitting boxes', pp. 85–86.

36 Amanda Gardner, 'FDA Panel Calls for Strongest Warning on ADHD Drugs', *Healthday News*, 9 February 2006.

37 Ray Moynihan, 'Drug maker's powerful immunization', *Australian Financial Review,* 29 November 2002.

38 ibid.

39 ibid.

40 'Republican National Convention: George W. Bush Cements Nomination, Cheney Accepts Vice Presidential Nod; Ford Hospitalized', *Larry King Live,* Transcript, 3 August 2000. Available at http://transcripts.cnn.com/TRANSCRIPTS/0008/03/lkl.00.html (accessed 27 March 2008).

41 Sax, 'Ritalin: Better Living Through Chemistry?' (Sax quotes these statistics from Jodie Morse, 'Summertime and School Isn't Easy', *Time*, 31 July 2000, p. 20. French students scored 23 points above the international average; Japanese students, 94 points above. German students on average were 5 points below the international average; American students, 39 points below.

Chapter 5: The Politics of ADHD

1   Western Australia, *Parliamentary Debates,* Legislative Assembly, 22 October 1997, p. 7299 (Kevin Prince, Minister for Health).

2   Western Australia, *Parliamentary Debates,* Legislative Assembly, 27 September 2007, p. 5946 (Alan Carpenter, Premier).

3   National Health and Medical Research Council, *Attention Deficit Hyperactivity Disorder (ADHD),* Canberra, 1997, p. 32.

4   ibid., p. 34.

5   ibid., p. 38.

6   Health Minister Tony Abbott MHR, *ADHD Review,* media release, 2 May 2007.

7   The Royal Australasian College of Physicians, 'Trade Exhibition and Sponsorship', *Physicians Week 2009.* Available at http://www. physiciansweek.com/sponex.asp (accessed 12 August 2009).

8   Janet Fife-Yeomans, 'ADHD reviewer double-up', *The Daily Telegraph,* 30 April 2007. Available at http://www.dailytelegraph.com.au/news/ nsw-act/adhd-reviewer-double-up/story-e6freuzi-1111113435833 (accessed 21 September 2008).

9   ibid.

10   Janet Fife-Yeomans, 'ADHD guru quits over Ritalin link', *The Daily Telegraph,* 5 May 2007. Available at http://www.dailytelegraph. com.au/news/nsw-act/adhd-guru-quits-over-ritalin-link/ story-e6freuzi-1111113472188.

11   Janet Fife-Yeomans and Bruce McDougall, 'As one boy enjoys life without medication, experts ask – Why do we drug our children?', *The Daily Telegraph,* 27 April 2007.

12   Janet Fife-Yeomans, 'ADHD guru quits over Ritalin link'.

13   'Call for policy on ADHD drugs', *Courier-Mail,* 27 April 2007.

14   Janet Fife-Yeomans, 'Secrecy for ADHD doctors', *The Daily Telegraph,* 30 June 2007.

15   Janet Fife-Yeomans, 'Guidelines panel linked to drug firms', *The Advertiser,* 17 November 2008, Available at http://www.news.com.au/ adelaidenow/story/0,22606,24660999-5006301,00.html (accessed 4 October 2009).

16   ibid.

17   ibid.

18   Commonwealth of Australia, *Parliamentary Debates,* Senate, 27 November 2008, p. 7540 (Senator Joe Ludwig on behalf of Hon Nicola Roxon, Minister for Health and Ageing).

19   Fife-Yeomans and McDougall, 'Call for ADHD drug inquiry'.

20 ibid.

21 Fife-Yeomans and McDougall, 'As one boy enjoys life without medication, experts ask – Why do we drug our children?'

22 Fife-Yeomans, 'Guidelines panel linked to drug firms'.

23 NHMRC, 'Draft Australian Guidelines on ADHD – NHMRC consideration deferred pending outcome of USA investigation', NHMRC Noticeboard 2009. Available at http://www.nhmrc.gov.au/media/noticeboard/notice09/091130-adhd.htm (accessed 5 January 2010).

24 Renee Viellaris, 'Medication not first option to beat ADHD', *Courier-Mail*, 1 December 2009.

25 This figure comes from M. G. Sawyer, F. M. Arney et al., 'The mental health of young people in "Australia: key findings from the child and adolescent component of the national survey of mental health and well-being', *Australian and New Zealand Journal of Psychiatry*, 35:806–814, 2001.

26 Statistics on number of patients on Attention Deficit Hyperactivity Disorder (ADHD) drugs in 2007 obtained through *Freedom of Information Act 1992*.

27 *Draft ADHD Guidelines Released*, Joint Media Release, 30 November 2009. The Hon Nicola Roxon MP, Minister for Health and Ageing, National Health and Medical Research Council, and Royal Australasian College of Physicians.

28 Kate Sikora, 'ADHD guidelines pulled after payment scandal', *The Daily Telegraph*, 23 November 2009.

29 Nicola Berkovic, 'Review of "tainted" ADHD guidelines', *The Australian*, 24 November 2009.

30 Harris and Carey, 'Researchers Fail to Reveal Full Drug Pay'.

31 'The Evolving Face of ADHD: From Adolescence to Adulthood—Clinical Implications'. Available at www.adhdhome.com (accessed 2 May 2008).

32 Gardiner Harris, '3 Researchers at Harvard are named in subpoena', *The New York Times*, 27 March 2009.

33 Emily Ramshaw, 'University of Texas officials vow to strengthen ethics rules for researchers', *The Dallas Morning News*, 11 February 2009.

34 Greg Birnbaum and Douglas Montaro, 'Shrinks for Sale. Analyze This: Docs get Drug Co. $$', *New York Sunday Post*, 28 February 1999.

35 Associated Press, 'Study Warns of Ritalin Side Effects in Preschoolers', 19 October 2006. Available at http://www.foxnews.com/story/0,2933,222559,00.html (accessed 25 July 2008).

36 International Association for Child and Adolescent Psychiatry and Allied Professions (IACAPAP) September 2006 Conference Melbourne Australia.

37 Royal Australasian College of Physicians, 'Draft Australian Guidelines on Attention Deficit Hyperactivity Disorder (ADHD)', p. 82.

38 M. S. McDonagh, K. Peterson, T. Dana, S. Thakurta, 'Drug Class Review on Pharmacologic Treatments for ADHD'. 2007. Available at http://www.ohsu.edu/drugeffectiveness/reports/final.cfm (accessed 13 February 2009).

39 Royal Australasian College of Physicians, 'Draft Australian Guidelines on Attention Deficit Hyperactivity Disorder (ADHD)', p. xviii.

40 ibid.

41 ibid., p. xxi.

42 Julie-Anne Davies, 'Probe into anti-depressants being conducted "in secret"', *The Australian*, 1 November 2008.

43 Ritalin (R) LA: methylphenidate hydrochloride, *Consumer Medicine Information*, March 2007. Available at http://www.nps.org.au/__data/assets/pdf_file/0011/16004/nvcrtlla10307.pdf (accessed 29 June 2009).

44 Royal Australasian College of Physicians, 'Draft Australian Guidelines on Attention Deficit Hyperactivity Disorder (ADHD)', p. 8.

45 ibid., p. xxiii.

46 ibid., p. 87.

47 ibid., p. 122.

48 Breggin, *Talking Back to Ritalin*, p. 264.

49 ibid., p. 253.

50 Justine Ferrari, 'Alert over ADHD guidelines in schools', *The Australian*, 19 August 2008.

51 Royal Australasian College of Physicians, 'Draft Australian Guidelines on Attention Deficit Hyperactivity Disorder (ADHD)', p. xxviii.

52 ibid.

53 ibid., p. 54.

54 ibid., p. xxi.

55 American Psychiatric Association, *Diagnostic and Statistical Manual of Mental Disorders*, Fourth Edition, pp. 92–93.

56 An ADHD diagnosis is usually sufficient but does not automatically guarantee the allowance. Parents must show the child 'has a physical, intellectual or psychiatric disability (that impacts on the family) and is likely to suffer from the disability permanently or for an extended period (that is, for 12 months or more)' Source: email received from Centrelink on 5 February 2008.

57 Graham, 'Drugs, labels and (p)ill–fitting boxes' p. 97.
58 In most states except Queensland GPs can't initiate treatment for
ADHD with stimulants.

Chapter 6: The Rise and Fall of ADHD in Western Australia

1 While there is no way of knowing for sure, the 85–90 per cent
proportion estimation may have been an overestimation. It was based
on the proportion of children in the ADHD prescription cohort
in New South Wales. A more conservative estimation of 70 per
cent would have meant there were approximately 14,600 Western
Australian children prescribed ADHD stimulants in 2000.
2 Government of Western Australia, Department of Health, *Attentional
Problems in Children: Diagnosis and Management of Attention Deficit
Hyperactivity Disorder (ADHD) and Associated Disorders,* Office of Mental
Health, Department of Health, Perth, 2002, p. 21.
3 Government of Western Australia, Department of Health,
Western Australian Stimulant Regulatory Scheme 2005 Annual Report,
Pharmaceutical Services Branch, Environmental Health Directorate,
Department of Health, Perth, 2006, p. iii.
4 Government of Western Australia, Department of Health,
Western Australian Stimulant Regulatory Scheme 2008 Annual Report,
Pharmaceutical Services Branch, Health Protection Group,
Department of Health, Perth, 2009, p. v.
5 Figure of 58 per cent obtained from statistical data supplied by
Government of Western Australia, Drug and Alcohol Office, via
email on 23 November 2009. Information supplied from draft 2008
report of *Australian School Student Survey 2008,* Table 18: Percentage of
students using non-prescribed amphetamine-like drugs in 2008 by age
and gender.
6 Until August 2005 dexamphetamine was the only drug for ADHD
subsidised through the Pharmaceutical Benefits Scheme (PBS). From
1993 until 2003, according to PBS data, WA was consistently the
highest prescribing state (or territory) for dexamphetamine. In 2003
the number of prescriptions dispensed for dexamphetamine was
around three and a half times higher per 1000 population than the
Australian average (including WA). In 2003, WA dispensed 86,980
prescriptions for dexamphetamine (WA pop. = 1,969,046) compared
to 61,390 in NSW (pop = 6,716,277) which was 44.2 prescriptions
per 1000 pop. in WA compared to NSW at 9.1 per 1000 and the
Australian average 12.5 per 1000. Department of Parliamentary

Services, *Medication for Attention Deficit/Hyperactivity Disorder (ADHD): an Analysis by Federal Electorate (2001-03),* Current Issues Brief. 16 November 2004, No. 8 2004-2005, Parliament of Australia, p. 7.

7   While Australian per capita consumption rates of stimulant medication were lower than US and Canadian rates, between 1994 and 2000 the per capita rates for the use of psychostimulants in WA were similar in the US and Canada. Constantine G. Berbatis, V. Bruce Sunderland et al., 'Licit psychostimulant consumption in Australia', p. 539.

8   Professor Trevor Parry, *Inquiry into Attention Deficit Disorder and Attention Deficit Hyperactivity Disorder in Western Australia,* Transcript of Evidence taken at Perth, Friday 20 August 2004, Education and Health Standing Committee, p. 5.

9   South Australian ADHD prescribing rates were second only to Western Australia's throughout the 1990s. They grew in the 1990s, until 1999 when Nash moved to Perth; then they continued to fall until Dr Nash returned to Adelaide in 2001. *36th Parliament Education and Health Standing Committee Report,* No. 8 'ADHD in WA', p. 18. Available at http://www.parliament.wa.gov.au/Parliament/commit.nsf/ (Report+Lookup+by+Com+ID)/085DC33FBCF9099348256F47002 4E396/$file/ADD+final+report+pdf+version.pdf (accessed 20 August 2009).

10   *Sixty Minutes* 'Out of control Sunday', 25 September 2005. Available at http://sixtyminutes.ninemsn.com.au/article.aspx?id=259344 (accessed 26 June 2009).

11   Ferguson and Rushworth, 'ADHD – the quick fix'.

12   Professor Trevor Parry, *Inquiry into Attention Deficit Disorder and Attention Deficit Hyperactivity Disorder in Western Australia,* p. 5.

13   Dr Trevor Parry, quoted in George Halasz, et al., 'Smartening up or dumbing down?: A Look Behind the Symptoms, Overprescribing and Reconceptualizing ADHD', *Cries unheard: a new look at attention deficit hyperactivity disorder,* Altona Vic, Common Ground Publishing 2002, p. 80.

14   ibid.

15   Western Australia Legislative Assembly, *Attention Deficit Hyperactivity Disorder in Western Australia,* Education and Health Standing Committee, Report No. 8, 2004, p. 23.

16   Western Australian Government, Department of Health, *Western Australian Stimulant Regulatory Scheme 2005 Annual Report,* Pharmaceutical Services Branch, Environmental Health Directorate,

Department of Health, Perth, 2006.

17   Western Australian Government, Department of Health, *Western Australian Stimulant Regulatory Scheme 2008 Annual Report*, Pharmaceutical Services Branch, Health Protection Group, Department of Health, Perth, 2009.

18   'The parent is frequently the sole source of information and often educational and behavioural information is not sought. When information is sought from the school, the questions asked are frequently inappropriate. Behavioural observations are rarely obtained.' *The Report of the Technical Working Party on Attention Deficit Disorder to the Cabinet Sub-Committee*, Parliament House Western Australia, 1997, p. 8.

19   ibid., p. 2.

20   ibid., p. 4.

21   ibid., p. 6.

22   ibid., p. 20.

23   ibid.

24   WA Stimulants Minutes 20 February 2002, obtained through *Freedom of Information Act 1992*.

25   The term mg/kg refers to recommended dose in milligrams of medication per kilogram of body weight.

26   WA Stimulants Minutes 20 February 2002, obtained under Freedom of Information Act 1992.

27   WA Stimulants Committee Minutes 10 November 1998, obtained through *Freedom of Information Act 1992*.

28   WA Stimulants Committee Minutes 2 November 1999 ,obtained through *Freedom of Information Act 1992*.

29   WA Stimulants Committee Minutes 26 September 2001, obtained through *Freedom of Information Act 1992*; WA Stimulants Committee Minutes 20 February 2002, obtained through *Freedom of Information Act 1992*.

30   WA Stimulants Committee Minutes on 20 February 2002, obtained under *Freedom of Information Act 1992*.

31   WA Stimulants Committee Minutes 21 August 2002, obtained under *Freedom of Information Act 1992*.

32   Wendy Pryer, 'Dismay at child attention disorder figures', *The West Australian*, 1 September 1999.

33   *Medical.WA Forum*, 'WA GPs surveyed – surprising results', Press Release – Health Reporter, 28 April 2006. Available at http://www.medicalhub.com.au/index.php?option=com_docman&task=doc_download&gid=84 (accessed 9 July 2009).

34 *The Report of the Technical Working Party on Attention Deficit Disorder to the Cabinet Sub-Committee*, p. 5.

35 Statistics obtained from the Medicare Australia website, relating to the prescription of stimulant medications, show that in WA 11,338 prescriptions for stimulant medication were subsidised by the PBS in 1994. By 1999, this figure had risen to 68,869. Available at https://www.medicareaustralia.gov.au/statistics/pbs_item.shtml.

36 Martin Whitely MLA, 'Inaugural speech', *Hansard,* Parliament of Western Australia, Thursday 3 May 2001, pp. 152b–179a.

37 Every prescriber was compelled to 'apply to the (West Australian) Department of Health and obtain a unique Stimulant Prescriber Number (SPN) to initiate stimulant treatment in any patient. The practitioner must provide individual patient details, including age, gender and dose required, thus enabling the collection of data for future analysis of stimulant use in WA'. Education and Health Standing Committee, Attention Deficit Hyperactivity Disorder in Western Australia, Report No. 8, 36th Parliament of Western Australia, October 2004, p. 27.

38 Amanda James, 'WA top State for "Dexies"', *The West Australian,* 24 September 2002.

39 *Attentional Problems in Children: Diagnosis and Management of Attention Deficit Hyperactivity Disorder (ADHD) and Associated Disorders*, p. 21.

40 Government of Western Australia, Department of Health, *Western Australian Stimulant Regulatory Scheme 2005 Annual Report,* Pharmaceutical Services Branch, Environmental Health Directorate, Department of Health, Perth, 2006, p. iii.

41 Government of Western Australia, Department of Health, *Western Australian Stimulant Regulatory Scheme 2008 Annual Report,* Pharmaceutical Services Branch, Health Protection Group, Department of Health, Perth, 2009.

42 Government of Western Australia, Department of Health, *Stimulant Prescribing and Usage Patterns for the Treatment of ADHD in Western Australia – 1 August 2003 to 31 December 2004,* Pharmaceutical Services Branch, Department of Health, Perth, 2005, p. v.

Conclusion: Where to From Here?

1 Martin Whitely, *Western Australian Parliamentary Debates*, Legislative Assembly, 3 May 2001, p 158 / 1.

2 Martin Whitely, *Western Australian Parliamentary Debates*, Legislative Assembly, 8 March 2006, pp 138b–176b / 2

Appendix 1: Strattera's Sad Short Story

1 G. Chouinard, L. Annable, and J. Bradwejn, 'An early phase II clinical trial of tomoxetine (LY139603) in the treatment of newly admitted depressed patients', *Psychopharmacology,* 83, 1984, p. 126.

2 Letter to Martin Whitely MLA from Eli Lilly Australia Pty Ltd, 1 December 2009.

3 David Michelson, Douglas Faries, et al., 'Atomoxetine in the Treatment of Children and Adolescents with Attention-Deficit/ Hyperactivity Disorder: A Randomized, Placebo-controlled, Dose-response study', *Pediatrics,* Vol. 108, No. 5, November 2001. Available at http://pediatrics.aappublications.org/cgi/content/full/108/5/e83 (accessed 13 January 2008).

4 ibid.

5 ibid.

6 ibid.

7 ibid.

8 Eli Lilly Website, http://www.strattera.com/1_3_childhood_adhd/1_3_1_1_what_is.jsp (accessed 14 January 2008, now removed from site).

9 Lilly advertisement for Strattera, appeared in *US News & World Report,* 26 April 2004, p. 65.

10 Food and Drug Administration, Letter to Eli Lilly and Company, Division of Drug Marketing, Advertising, and Communications, Food and Drug Administration, Maryland, June 2005. Available at http://www.pharmcast.com/WarningLetters/Yr2005/Jun2005/EliLilly0605.htm (accessed 23 September 2008).

11 Liz Tickner, 'Drug to cut schoolyard trade', *The West Australian,* 16 April 2004.

12 Charlie Wilson-Clark, 'Aid for new ADHD drug sought', *The West Australian,* 17 April 2004.

13 Kylie Walker, 'New drug combats child addiction fears', *Courier-Mail,* 15 April 2004.

14 Ben Wyld, 'Milder new drug hailed for attention disorder', *The Sydney Morning Herald,* 15 April 2004.

15 Martin Whitely, *Western Australian Parliamentary Debates*, Legislative Assembly, 23 November 2006, page 8772b – 8774a / 1.

16 Food and Drug Administration, *Warning on Liver Injury from Strattera: FDA Patient Safety News: Show #37,* March 2005. Available at http://www.accessdata.fda.gov/psn/printer.cfm?id=302 (accessed 18 July 2007).

17 US Food and Drug Administration, *Public Health Advisory: Suicidal Thinking in Children and Adolescents Being Treated with Strattera (Atomoxetine),* 17 December 2004. Available at http://www.fda. gov./Drugs/DrugSafety/PublicHealthAdvisories/ucm051733.htm (accessed 13 September 2009); 'In the review of 2,200 patients, 1,357 of whom were taking Strattera, researchers found that 0.4 percent of the children taking the drug reported suicidal thinking, compared to no cases in children taking a placebo. There was also one suicide attempt in the Strattera group.' Amanda Gardner, 'FDA Issues Alert on ADHD Drug Strattera', *Healthday Reporter,* September 29 2005. Available at http://psychdata.blogspot.com/2005/10/fda-issues-alert-on-adhd-drug.html (accessed 19 May 2010).

18 US Food and Drug Administration, *New Warning for Strattera,* Talk Paper, 17 December 2004. Available at: http://www.fda.gov/bbs/topics/ANSWERS/2004/ANS01335.html (accessed 11 April 2009).

19 Cathy O'Leary, 'WA kids still biggest users of ADHD pills', *The West Australian,* 1 October 2005.

20 Clara Pirani, 'The Dark Side of a Wonder Drug', *The Australian,* 28 March 2006.

21 Western Australia, *Parliamentary Debates,* Legislative Assembly, 23 November 2006: p. 8772 (Martin Whitely).

22 Quoted in WA 36th Parliament, Mr. M. P. Whitely [9.39 am] Thursday, 23 November 2006.

23 In 2003 I was instrumental in helping to establish Drug Free Attention Difficulties Support (DFADS) designed to achieve two objectives. First to influence public policy as it relates to ADHD and second to provide support to parents and patients who wish to try drug-free approaches.

24 Adverse events information related to Strattera obtained from the Therapeutic Goods Administration's Public Case Detail reports.

25 A 2008 study by Curtin University pharmacologist Con Berbatis identified that, because reporting is voluntary, only a tiny fraction (for GPs only 2 per cent) of adverse event is reported. Con Berbatis, 'Primary care and Pharmacy: 4. Large contributions to national

adverse reaction reporting by pharmacists in Australia', *i2P E-Magazine*, Issue 72, June 2008.

26 Government of Western Australia, *Inquiry into Attention Deficit Disorder and Attention Deficit Hyperactivity Disorder in Western Australia*, Legislative Assembly, Transcript of evidence taken on 16 June 2004, pp. 8-9 (Associate Professor Heather Jenkins).

27 Letter from Curtin University to Office of the Information Commissioner in response to MW application, dated 14 September 2007, p. 6.

28 *Information for Parents about Strattera*, p. 1, n.d., obtained through *Freedom of Information Act 1992*.

29 Julie-Anne Davies, 'Curtin University misled about ADHD drug', *The Australian*, January 10 2009. Available at http://www.theaustralian. news.com.au/story/0,25197,24893755-12332,00.html (accessed 24 June 2009).

30 ibid.

31 ibid.

32 ibid. Note: Associate Professor Jenkins appears to have cited the incorrect publication she used to support her incorrect claim to the ethics committee that the FDA had revoked the Strattera warning. According to a summary document provided by Curtin University that details Professor Jenkins's argument, she said it had appeared in the *Harvard Mental Health Letter* in April 2006. No such article appeared in that issue but an article by the same name and by the same author does appear in the April 2006 edition of *Pediatric News*.

33 ibid.

34 ibid.

35 ibid.

36 ibid.

37 Julie Robotham, 'New drug can make children suicidal', *The Sydney Morning Herald*, 8 December 2006.

Appendix 2: Sydney Repeats Perth's Mistakes

1   Janet Fife-Yeomans, 'The Ritalin Generation – Top judge condemns the ADHD explosion', *The Daily Telegraph*, 26 April 2007.

2   ibid.

3   Clinical Excellence Commission, *Attention Deficit Hyperactivity Disorder in Children and Adolescents in New South Wales – 2007: Final Report of the Special Review*, Sydney, December 2007, p. 64. Available at http:// www.cec.health.nsw.gov.au/pdf/specialreports/adhd_080211.pdf (accessed 31 August 2009).

4 ibid., pp. 64–65.
5 ibid., p. 32.
6 ibid., p. 20.
7 ibid., p. 25.
8 ibid., p. 15; Allegra Stratton, 'Questions raised about drugs as treatment for ADHD sufferers' *The Guardian*, 12 November 2007.
9 Clinical Excellence Commission, *Attention Deficit Hyperactivity Disorder in Children and Adolescents in New South Wales – 2007*, p. 24.
10 'For 7% of practices, patients with this condition (ADHD) comprised 51-90% of their patients and for one practice (0.5% of the sample) having patients with this condition accounted for more than 90% of their patients.' ibid., p. 20.
11 '34% of paediatricians, and only 5% of child psychiatrists, prescribing to 100 or more patients.' ibid., p. 27.
12 ibid., p. 32.
13 Janet Fife-Yeomans, 'Go sit in the corner – Judge who spoke out against Ritalin kids gagged', *The Daily Telegraph,* 25 February 2008.
14 In 2003, WA dispensed 86,980 prescriptions for dexamphetamine (WA pop = 1,969, 046) compared to 61,390 in NSW (pop = 6,716,277) which was 44.2 prescriptions per 1000 pop in WA compared to NSW at 9.1/1000 and the Australian average 12.5/1000. Department of Parliamentary Services, *Medication for Attention Deficit/Hyperactivity Disorder (ADHD): an Analysis by Federal Electorate (2001-03),* Current Issues Brief 16 November 2004, No. 8 2004–2005, Parliament of Australia, Canberra, p. 7.
15 There were 15,466 boys and 3872 girls aged four to seventeen on ADHD medication in NSW in the survey period, between June 1 2006 and May 31 2007. Clinical Excellence Commission, *Attention Deficit Hyperactivity Disorder in Children and Adolescents in New South Wales – 2007*, p. 12. This meant approximately 0.28 per cent of the NSW population aged four to seventeen were on stimulant medication. There were 6188 Western Australian children (four to seventeen) on stimulants in the 2007 calendar year. Government of Western Australia, Department of Health, *Western Australian Stimulant Regulatory Scheme 2007 Annual Report,* Pharmaceutical Services Branch, Health Protection Group, Department of Health, Perth, 2008, p. 41. This meant approximately 0.29 per cent of the WA population aged four to seventeen were on stimulant medication. Note: NSW population 6,926,990, WA 2,130,797. Australian Bureau of Statistics Population, Australian States and Territories, December 2007.

16 For NSW from 1 July 2006 to 31 May 2007 there were 75,932 scripts
and from 1 July 2008 to 30 June 2009 there were 170,634 scripts for
ADHD drugs subsidised by the PBS. For WA from 1 January 2007 to
31 December 2007, there were 67,202 scripts and from 1 July 2008 to
30 June 2009 there were 77,305 scripts for ADHD drugs subsidised
by the PBS. Source Medicare Australia website self-generated report
prepared by Martin Whitely on 29 August 2009 using https://www.
medicareaustralia.gov.au/statistics/pbs_item.shtml; Since 2007 new
drugs including Strattera, Concerta and Ritalin LA were added to the
PBS which may account for part or all of the increase in WA, however,
not for the massively disproportionate growth in NSW.

Further Reading

Baughman Jr MD., F. A., and Hovey, C., *The ADHD Fraud: How Psychiatry Makes 'Patients' of Normal Children*, Trafford Publishing, Victoria BC, 2006.

Breggin, MD., P. R., *Talking Back to Ritalin: What Doctors Aren't Telling You about Stimulants for Children,* Common Courage Press, Monroe, 1998.

Jacobs, B., Youth Affairs Network of Queensland, *Being an Educated Consumer of 'ADHD' Research*, Youth Affairs Network of Queensland, 2005.

Moynihan. R. and Cassels, A., *Selling Sickness: How the World's Biggest Pharmaceutical Companies Are Turning us all into Patients,* Nation Books, New York, 2005.

Timimi, S, et al., 'A Critique of the International Consensus Statement on ADHD', *Clinical Child and Family Psychology Review,* Vol. 7, No. 1, 2004.

Western Australian Legislative Assembly, *Attention Deficit Hyperactivity Disorder in Western Australia,* Education and Health Standing Committee, Report No. 8, 2004.

Acknowledgments

Martin Whitely acknowledges the ethical professionalism of psychiatrists like Dr Peter Breggin (USA), Dr Sami Timimi (UK), Dr Jon Jureidini and Dr George Halasz (Australia) who have been prepared to swim against the tide of money and misinformation that has swamped too many of their colleagues.

Martin also acknowledges the efforts of mothers like Sue Saltmarsh, Katherine Frances and Juie Greatbatch who have fought for the rights and welfare of not just their own children, but all children.

Martin also thanks Kim Heitman, Director of Legal Services at The University of Western Australia, for legal advice in regards to the contents of this book.

Finally Martin acknowledges Melinda, Shane and Patrick for tolerating his 'deficit of attention' on the home front for the years it took to write *Speed Up and Sit Still*.

Index